Best wishes
Nora McNamara

Who Brings Trees Brings Life
People and Trees in Igalaland

Sr. Nora McNamara
Dr. Stephen Morse

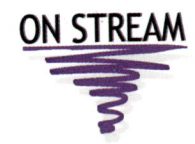

ON STREAM

Published 2004 by Onstream Publications Ltd.
Currabaha, Cloghroe, Co Cork, Ireland
info@onstream.ie

© Sr Nora McNamara & Dr Stephen Morse.

ISBN: 1897 685 73 4

For Onstream:
Editor: Roz Crowley
Design: Nick Sanquest
Printing: Betaprint Ltd., Dublin

Editor (Reading) Erika Meller
Artist: Henry A. Adama
Photographs: Clement Agada, Moses Acholo.

Botanical Information adapted from J.Hutchinson and J.M.Dalziel
'Flora of West Tropical Africa'
volumes 1 to 3; Crown Agents, London

No part of this book may be reproduced in any form without permission in writing from the publisher.

•Contributors

Daniel Acholo
Moses Acholo
Clement Agada
Babatunde Akinsinde
Benjamin Daramola
Raymond Emere
Uche Ezeama
Bernard Ezeama
Ken Friedman
Mrs L Holis-Kim
Daniel Ibrahim
Paul Idrisu
Remigius Ikkah
Daniel Jekelyi
Vincent Neussl
Isaac Obaka
Gerard Obaje
Catherine Oguonu
Chief Philip Okwoli
Abdullahi Ocholo
Sunday Onakpa
Stephen Okanebu
Ambrose Salifu
Idrisu Sule
Terimu Usman
Chris Vassiliu
Andrew Ward

Foreword by His Royal Highness the Attah of Igala

This book is a compendium of trees in the Igala Kingdom. It is good to know the importance of trees and their fruits in our society.

It is a pleasure for me, therefore, to write a foreword to this book on the People and Trees of Igalaland. The challenge before Igala sons and daughters is that they should know the importance of trees in their surroundings. Wood from trees is used to roof our houses and for making our furniture. Some fruits of these trees are edible and nourish our bodies. The leaves, roots and skin of these trees can also be used to cure some ailments. My own favourite tree is the mango.

I congratulate the contributors and authors most sincerely for their efforts. This book will serve as an inspiration to others who have positive contributions to make for the upliftment of Igalaland.

Alhaji (Dr) Aliyu O. Obaje
CBE, CON, FIAMN, LLD, CFR
ATTAH IGALA

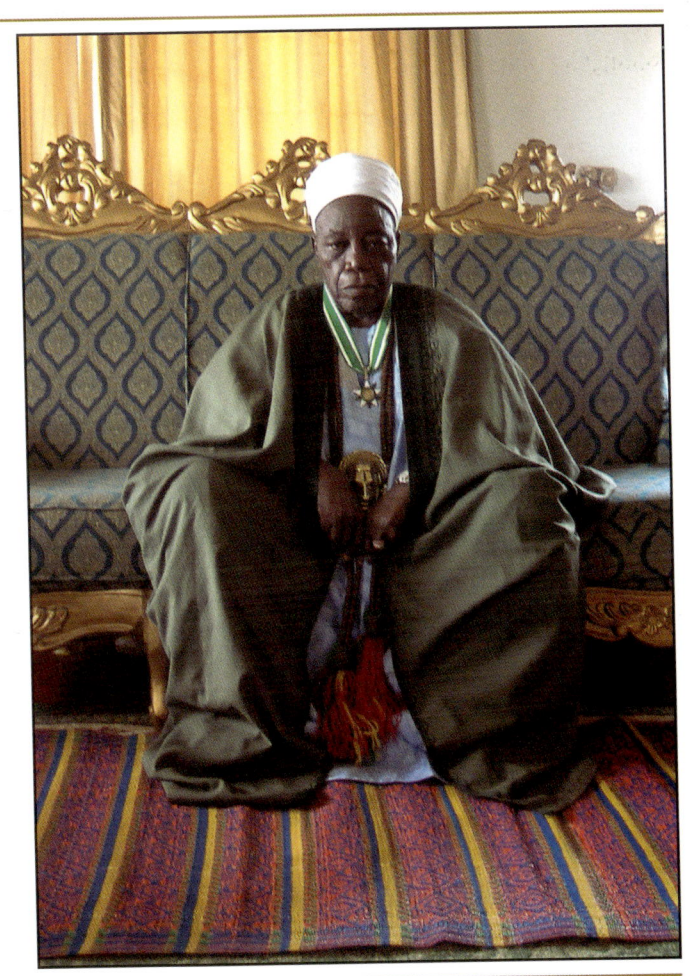

•Introduction

The trees of Igala have many messages for us and on their behalf we need to express concern for trees worldwide. Foremost in their communiqués comes fear of extinction of other indigenous trees which can trigger further climatic changes, declining soil fertility and subsequent threats to food sources.

The purpose of Who Brings Trees Brings Life is to provide practical insights into the current condition of trees in Igalaland Kogi State, Nigeria and how they can best be utilized. Fortunately there still exists local knowledge about trees and this needs to be recorded before its custodians pass away. This book catalogues information on 50 trees to allow their multiplicity of uses to be celebrated into the future. Information further needs to be recorded on the other 250 trees identified in the course of this study, if the celebration is to be on-going.

Many important lessons have been learned in the course of our investigation which confirmed fears that farmers and growers have made known over the years. These often refer to tree species cleared for farming, housing and export, which have not been replaced. Hitherto such trees were naturally regenerated in the wild and required no maintenance. This is no longer true and means there is currently a lack of knowledge of how these trees are grown which makes research and networking of the utmost importance in the coming years. This study also looks at trees which will continue to play a key role in the well being of Igala society in the future. To the forefront of these are oil palm, raphia palm, coconut, orange and fuel woods. Some of these trees were seriously endangered from the 1970s onwards, but thanks to the wisdom of the farmers who sought information on maintenance, considerable work in the region was possible. Others like *gmelina* were barely known. Fruits such as oranges and pawpaw were scarce.

But the situation has changed, thanks to Gorta, an Irish partner concerned with the eradication of famine and which views trees as critical to this goal. It has been helping the Diocesan Development Services (DDS) since the mid 1970s when oil palm maintenance was viewed by farmers as central to their survival. Oil palm is the premier cash crop in the locality and the main ingredient in most meals and health care.

With good advice on maintenance, trees have helped the economy, and nurseries where seedlings could be produced further enhanced the situations of many farmers. Another important event which gave impetus to this particular work was the recognition by the communities that their land was 'dying'. DDS had long recognised this as a serious issue, but it was only when individuals saw the disappearance of certain 'fertilizer trees' that something more concrete could be done. It was fortuitous that our quest for help with trees and their role in environmental and conservation issues coincided with that of scientists with similar pursuits.

These worked at ICRAF (International Centre for Research in Agroforestry, Nairobi, Kenya), which had a branch in Ibadan, Nigeria. There was a real meeting of minds between ICRAF and DDS which led to a breakthrough in DDS's work with trees. Because of Gorta's encouragement and funding it became possible to engage the services of Mr. Benjamin Daramola, a taxonomist, who identified the trees, their attributes and other relevant information contained here.

Together with Mr. Daramola and his colleague Mr. Babatunde Akinsinde, DDS travelled the length and breadth of Igalaland talking with farmers and housewives about how they perceived trees and their practical uses. It was very much a learning exercise, especially for the participants in our rustic areas. Their concerns about the disappearance of trees became only too apparent, in particular fuelwoods for the women and hardwoods for the men. The men bemoaned the disappearance of trees that hitherto were self-propagating and generated the biomass and nitrogen essential for crops. The shortage of firewood was so acute in some areas that economic fruit trees, even the oil palms, were being cut for firewood. At the end of this study it seemed imperative to fully document what still remained of indigenous information about trees, especially those central to the livelihoods of those residing in the region. By 2002 it was apparent to DDS that the schools lacked teaching materials required to make the children aware of the richness of the local flora. Even the textbooks for biology students in secondary schools could be enhanced by providing interesting facts about trees in the region, along with the possibility of resolving the problem of scarcity of specimens when it came to exams.

The tree species have been listed alphabetically with no ranking or status implied. The trees chosen were selected by Igalas, not by us. The level of knowledge held by many people was truly astounding, but unfortunately this is being lost in the younger generation. We are conscious that this is a rather humble beginning and very much unfinished. However, we hope that this is a prelude to future editions. We would like to stress that this is not primarily a botanical book, rather a story of the Igala people's engagement with their trees.

For each tree there are four headings - food, culture, medicine and other uses (firewood, furniture, building). The whole exercise of obtaining some closely guarded secrets made the study a real honour and a privilege as the relationship with trees is highly sacrosanct. One could not but admire the reason for guarding many secrets, which could not be disclosed, as such information wrongly used might be dangerous.

The study illustrates the profundity of their lives, including their worship, relationships, health, food and livelihoods. It also confirms the wholeness of traditional society, clearly demonstrating it not as something static, but a rather dynamic institution that slowly but organically accommodates not only new tree species but ideas as well. Evidence of such progress in the number of new trees making their debut in the region in the last couple of decades.

At this point we would like to make it clear that though the different recipes described here have been extensively tested by herbalists over many generations, they can be dangerous unless prepared under the guidance and direction of experienced and responsible herbalists. If prepared carelessly they can kill. The World Health Organisation has estimated that some 80% of the world's population is dependent on traditional treatments so they are included here simply to highlight the range of medicinal applications. However, this book is not intended to be a pharmacopia.

This work would have been impossible without the support and encouragement of Gorta. To them we are most grateful. Without this long-term relationship spanning some 30 years much of the environmental and conservation work would not have got off the ground. This book is therefore a tribute to Gorta.

We would also like to acknowledge the support of APSO, now part of Development Co-operation Ireland (DCI) and Trocaire for their roles. Our big thanks must go to Bishop E. S. Obot for his encouragement and appreciation. His Royal Highness the Attah of Igala also deserves a special word of thanks for promoting DDS projects. It is hoped that leadership of this calibre will help inspire love and appropriate action for the conservation and promotion of our trees.

Nora McNamara
Stephen Morse
Idah, August 2003

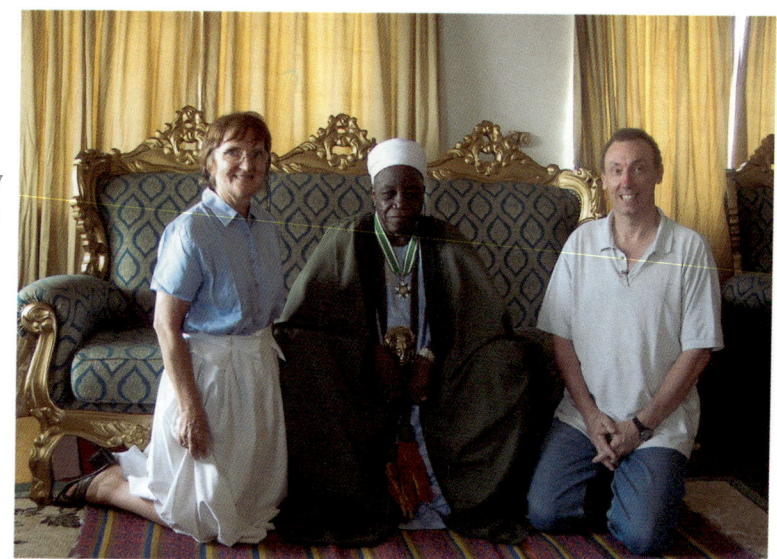

Foreword by the Bishop of Idah

As a spiritual leader, it is part of my responsibility to nurture and promote all that is good in creation.

> *"God looked at his work and saw that is was good."*
> (Gen. 1:31)

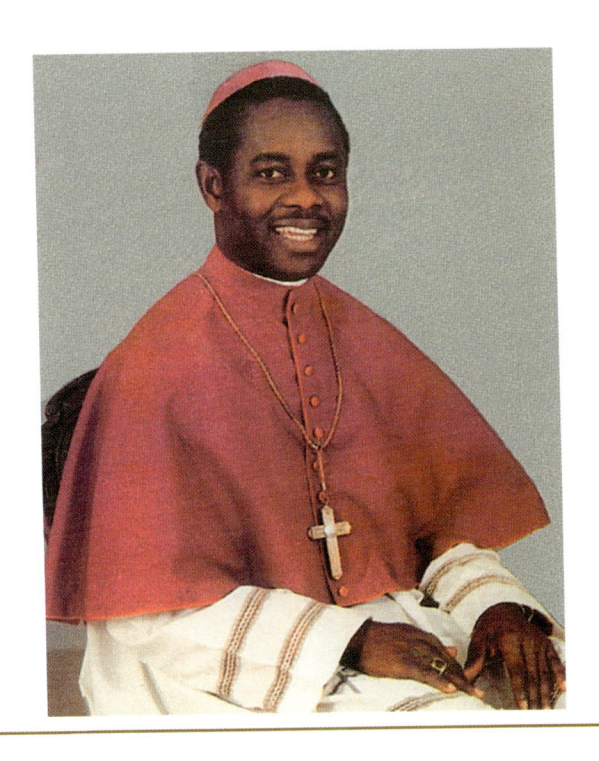

Trees have always been perceived as being part of the garden of Eden, so it is not surprising that every mission compound and all Church-run institutions have a collection of trees – ornamental, fruit or multi-purpose.

Nowadays we are all much more conscious of our environment and the damage it has been dealt by our affluence and the felling of trees. This study looks only at 50 trees though the taxonomist involved identified over 300 tree species in Igalaland, many of which are endangered. The findings therefore give us some clues as to how we can proceed with conserving our environment.

This work, however, is only a humble beginning and, due to financial constraints, it could not include every part of the diocese. Subsequent editions will be more inclusive. On this note, I encourage contributors and editors to keep up the work of documenting our rich heritage of trees and I also recommend it to partners concerned with environmental issues.

Most Rev. E.S. Obot,
Bishop of Idah

•Species List

Family	Botanical name and authority	Common name	Igala name ANKPA	Igala name DEKINA	Igala name IDAH	Igala name IBAJI
Bombacaceae	*Adansonia digitata L.*	Baobab	Obobo	Obobo	Obobo	Obobo
Caesalpinioidae	*Afzelia africana Smith ex. Pers.*	Cam wood	Anwa	Anwa	Anwa	Anwa
Anacardiaceae	*Annacardium occidentale L.*	Cashew	Ikachu	Ikachu	Ikachu	Ikachu
Loganiaceae	*Anthocleista nobilis G. Don*	Cabbage Tree	Odologwu	Odologwu	Odogwu	Odogwu
Mimisiodae	*Aubrevillea kerstingii (Harms) Pellegrin*		Udu	Udu	Udu	Udu
Meliaceae	*Azadiracta indica Juss*	Neem	Oli-Ọda	Oli-Ọda	Oli-Ọda	Oli-Ọda
Bombacaceae	*Bombax costatum Pellegr & Vuillet*	Kapok tree	Agwu	Agwugwu	Agwugwu	Agwugwu
Caricaceae	*Carica papaya L.*	Pawpaw	Echibakpa	Echibakpa	Echibakpa	Echibakpa
Sapotaceae	*Chrysophyllum albidum G. Don*	African cherry	Ẹhia	Ẹhia	Utẹ	Utiẹ
Rutaceae	*Citrus aurantium L.*	Orange	Alemu	Alemu	Alemu	Ulomu
Rutaceae	*Citrus x tangelo*	Tangerine orange	Alemu	Alemu	Alemu	Ulomu
Palmae	*Cocos nucifera L.*	Coconut	Unọba	Unọba	Unọba	Unọba
Sterculiaceae	*Cola acuminata Schott & Endl.*	Cola	Obi-Igala	Obi-Igala	Obi-Igala	Obi-Igala
Sterculiaceae	*Cola gigantea Brenan & Keay*	Cola	Ugo	Ugo	Ugo	Ugo/Ebenebe
Sterculiaceae	*Cola nitida (Vent) Endl*	Cola	Obi-Akechi	Obi-Akechi	Obi-Akechi/Atala	Atala
Caesalpiniaceae	*Cynometra vogelii Hook F.*	Indigo	Uri	Uli	Uli	Uli
Caesalpiniaceae	*Daniellia oliveri (Rolfe) Hotch & Dalz*	African Copaiba Balsam Tree, West African Gum Copal	Agba	Agba	Agba	Agba/Akpach
Caesalpiniaceae	*Dialium guineense Willd*	Velvet Tamarind	Agirigele	Ayigẹlẹ	Ayigẹlẹ	Ayigẹlẹ
Meliaceae	*Ekebergia senegalensis A. Juss*		Ọrachi	Ọrachi	Ọrachi	Ọrachi
Palmae	*Elaeis guinensis Jacq*	Oil palm	Ẹkpẹ	Ẹkpẹ	Ẹkpẹ	Ẹkpẹ
Papilionaceae	*Erythrina senegalensis DC*	Coral Flower	Achẹchẹ	Achẹchẹ	Achẹchẹ	Achẹchẹ
Moraceae	*Ficus capensis Thumb*	Fig tree	Ogbaikolo	Ugbakolo	Ugbakolo	Ọgbakolo
Moraceae	*Ficus thonningii Blume*	Chinese banyan, Malayan banyan, Indian laurel	Ọda/Ogbu	Ọda	Ọda	Ọda
Verbenaceae	*Gmelina arborea Roxb.*	Gmelina	Gmelina	Gmelina	Gmelina	Gmelina
Simaroubaceae	*Hannoa undulata Planch*		Odobala		Umopula	

| | | | Igala name ||||
Family	Botanical name and authority	Common name	ANKPA	DEKINA	IDAH	IBAJI
Euphorbiaceae	*Hymenocardia acida* Tul	Miombo Red-heart	Ẹnache	Ẹnache	Ẹnache	Ẹnache
Irvingiaceae	*Invingia gabonensis* (O. Rorke) Baill	Bush mango	Ọrọ-Egili	Ọrọ-Egili	Ọrọ-Egili	Ọrọ-Egili
Irvingiaceae	*Irvingia wombulu* Vermoesen	Okra tree	Ọrọ -Ayikpẹlẹ	Ọrọ -Ayikpẹlẹ	Ọrọ -Ayikpẹlẹ	Ọrọ -Ayikpẹlẹ
Meliaceae	*Khaya senegalensis* (Des) A. Juss	Mahogani	Ago	Ago	Ago	Ago
Bignoniaceae	*Kigelia africana* Benth	Sausage tree	Ebiẹ	Ebiẹ	Ebie/Unya	Unya
Apocynaceae	*Landolphia amoena* Hug	Abo	Abo	Abo	Abo	Abo
Anacardiaceae	*Lannea nigritana* (sc. Ellioh) Keay	Hog plum	Igogo	Ochikala	Echikala	Echikala
Ochnaceae	*Lophira lanceolata* Van Tiegr. Ex Keay	Iron tree	Okopi	Okopi	Okopi	Okopi
Anacardiaceae	*Mangifera indica* L.	Mango	Umagolo	Umagolo	Umagolo	Umagolo
Moraceae	*Milicia excelsa* (Welw) C. C. Berg	Iroko tree	Uroko	Uroko	Uroko	Uroko
Rubiaceae	*Mitragyna inermis* (Willd.) O. Kuntze		Ọtọchi	Ọtọchi	Ọtọchi	Ọtọchi
Rubiaceae	*Morinda lucida* Benth	Bonko fruit	Ogẹlẹ	Ogẹlẹ	Ogẹlẹ	Ogẹlẹ
Bignoniaceae	*Newbouldia laevis* (Baeuv) Seem	African Border Tree	Ogirichi	Ogichi	Ogichi	Ogichi
Mimosaceae	*Parkia biglobosa* (Jacq) Benth	African locust bean	Ugba	Ugba	Ugba	Ugba
Lauraceae	*Persea americana* Miller	Avocado pears	Ube Agiliki	Ube Agiliki	Ube Agiliki	Ube Agiliki
Euphorbiaceae	*Phyllanthus discoides* (Baill)	Makarara	Ode	Ode	Ode	Ode
Palmae	*Podococcus barteri* Mann & Wendl.	Fan palm	Odo	Odo	Odo	Odo
Mimosaceae	*Prosopsis africana* (Guill ex perr) Taub	Locust bean	Okpehie	Okpuye	Okpuye	Okpuye
Myrtaceae	*Psidium guajava* L.	Guava	Igwoba	Igwoba	Igwoba	Igwoba
Papilionaceae	*Pterocarpus erinaceus* Poir	Barwood, Kino	Ache	Ache	Ache	Ache
Papilionaceae	*Pterocarpus santalinoides* L'Her.	Rose wood	Igbẹgbẹ	Igbẹgbẹ	Igbẹgbẹ	Igbẹgbẹ
Palmae	*Raphia sp*	Raphia palm	Ẹkpe-ugala	Ẹkpe-ugala	Ẹkpe-ugala	Ẹkpe-ugala
Verbenaceae	*Tectona grandis* Linn.f.*Treculia africana*	Teak	Oli-are	Oli-are	Oli-are	Oli-are
Moraceae	Decne	African bread fruit, African bread nut	Abakwu	Ẹhiọ	Ẹhiọ	Ẹhiọ
Verbenaceae	*Vitex doniana* Sweet	Meru-Oak	Ejiji	Ejiji	Ejiji	Ejiji

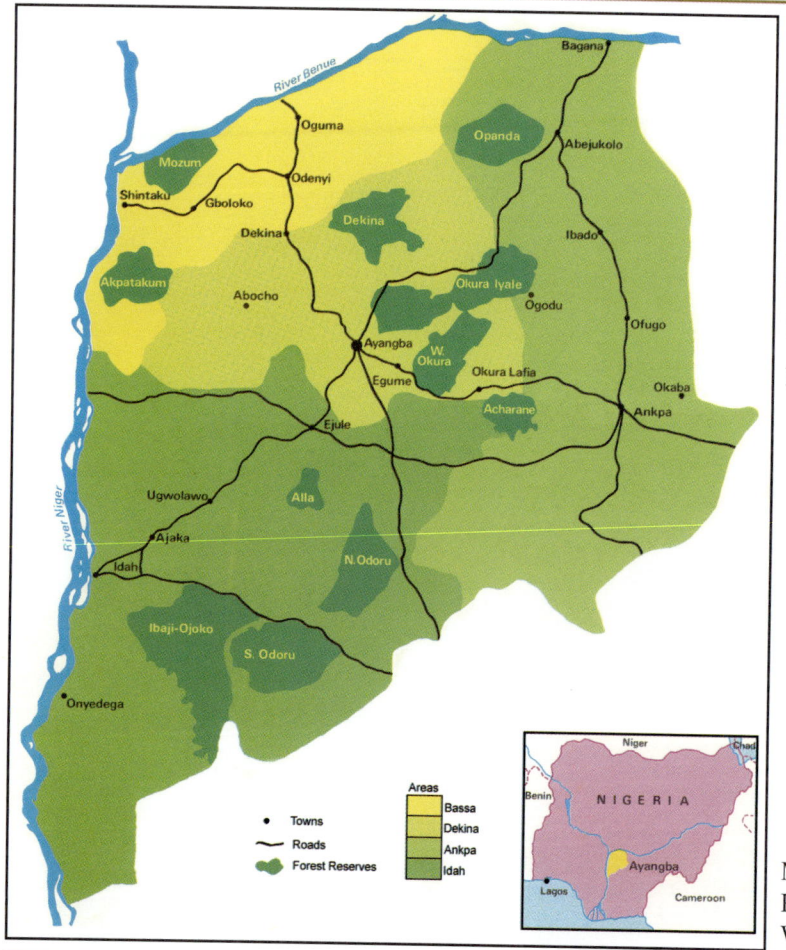

Map of Igala and Bassa lands showing the major towns and forest reserves.

Map adapted from: Ayangba Agricultural Development Project Extension Manual
World Bank, Washington.

Adansonia digitata

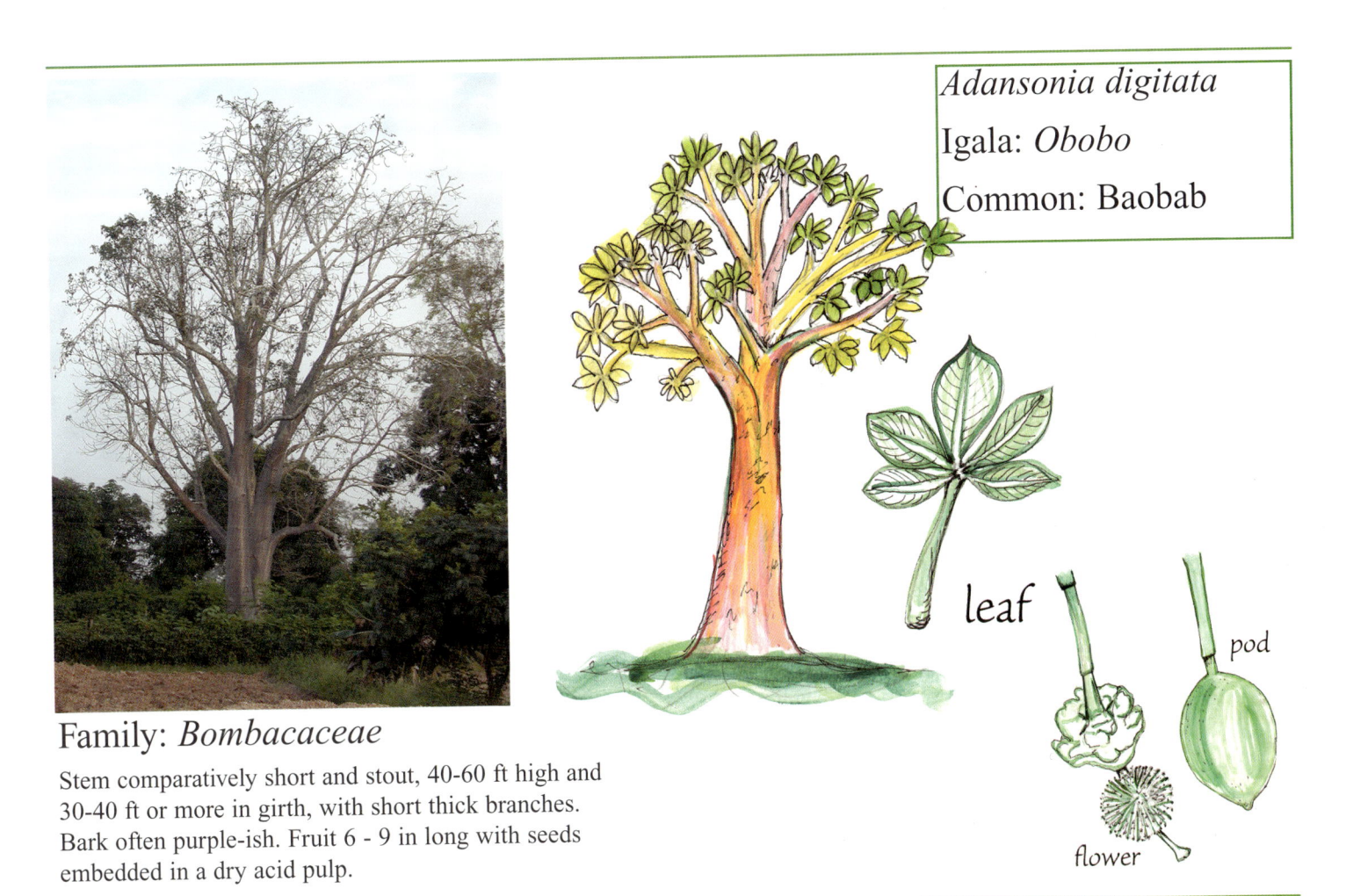

Igala: *Obobo*

Common: Baobab

Family: *Bombacaceae*

Stem comparatively short and stout, 40-60 ft high and 30-40 ft or more in girth, with short thick branches. Bark often purple-ish. Fruit 6 - 9 in long with seeds embedded in a dry acid pulp.

leaf

flower

pod

1

•Food

Children and adults lick the dried white part of the nut and find it refreshing and sweet.

Foodwise this tree has created a bond between the Hausa and Igala peoples and is a welcome symbol of cultural integration following many years of close contact between them. The leaves are ground into a paste, boiled with regular soup ingredients and eaten with *ojakpa*; this is the food of the Hausa people and now popular in Igalaland.

•Medicinal

Pregnant women use it to prevent oedema. A paste made from grinding the bark is applied all over the body before retiring.

For guinea worm sufferers the bark is also ground to a paste and applied externally. The bark and leaf can also be boiled and the liquid used to bathe; this helps draw the guinea worm to the surface of the skin.

The fruit when cooked cures malaria fever.

Picture shows a tree with bark removed for making local medicines.

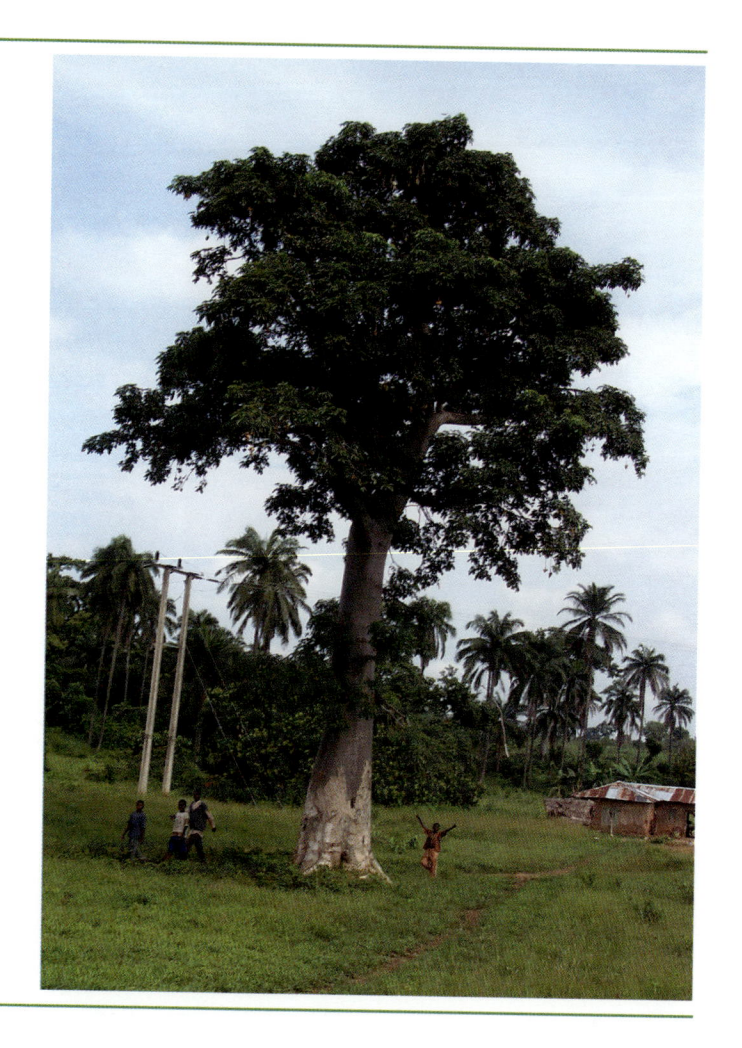

•Cultural

Masquerade heads are made from its wood.

It serves as a lightning conductor if positioned close to the house.

Igalas believe that a small iron axe (*Okanyi Akpabana*), known to be very dangerous, marks the spot where lightning strikes.

The baobab consumes the axe and therefore frees the area from lightning. The rainmakers know where to find such axes since they put them in a pot as part of the ceremony to attract rain.

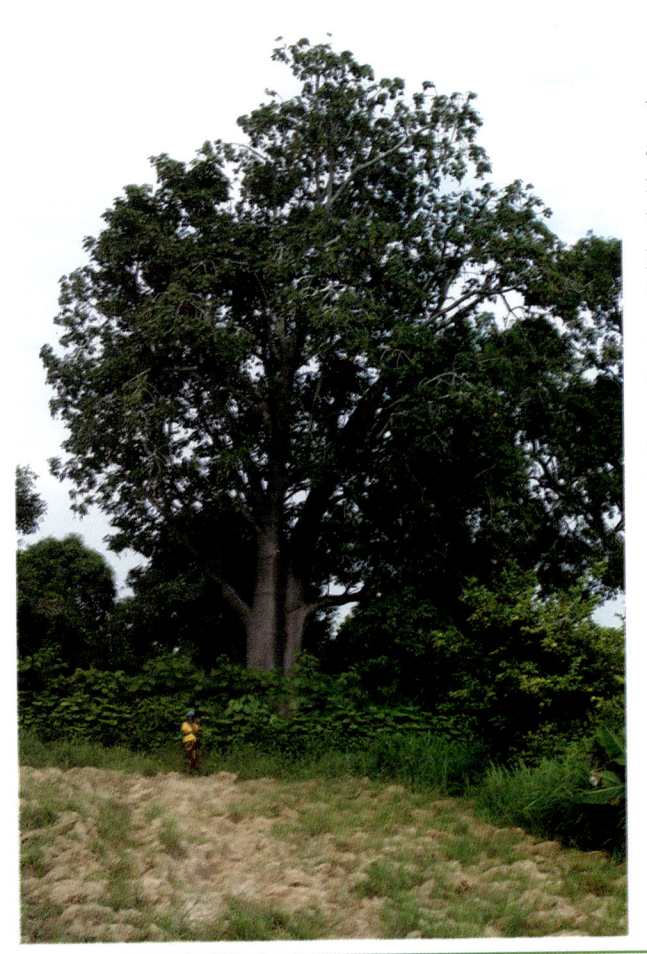

Very few are privy to the activities surrounding such rituals. However they are understood to be dangerous and parents warn their children about the dangers of touching the pot.

If touched, the axe will strike; and there has been a casualty with a rainmaker. The rainmaker in question went fishing and tried to prevent the rain from falling by using the ceremony, which included the axe.

Thunder struck immediately and he died instantly.

It is widely held that a mistake was made in some part of the ritual. Maybe the axe was turned in a wrong way; turned one way it brings rain, another it brings thunder, or the ceremony may have been incomplete.

Traditional knowledge relating to these ceremonies is closely guarded and not revealed because there is genuine fear the information may be misused.

Akpabana kpoli kpokwu kima kpobobo
Thunder and lightning can kill everything on earth but cannot kill baobab

•Other uses

The baobab is well recognized for helping maintain soil fertility, as the tree is turgid almost year round giving an abundance of leaves that decay easily.

Its shade protects the soil and cereal crops close to it grow well. It is high enough not to shade out a crop, yet low enough to give the protection they require, especially at the close of the rainy season when the scorching sun can destroy crops like maize.

Beneath this tree you will always find *Awolowo* grass (*Eupatorium odoratum*), a sure sign of good land. This is the case even if there has been no fallow period.

The baobab produces firewood which is long lasting. Its one drawback is that it dries very slowly.

It is never used for building of local houses because the (cuttings) sticks germinate.

It provides year round shade. So large are some trees that holes are sometimes made in its trunk allowing people to rest within its hollow to take respite from the hot sun.

Leaves are good for animal fodder.

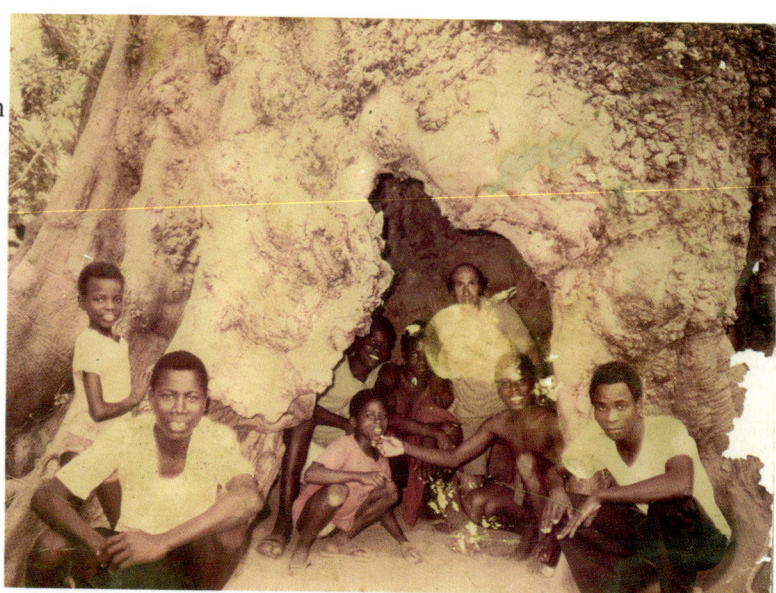

Rev. Fr Guertin and friends resting in a hollow baobab trunk.c.1968.

Afzelia africana
Igala: *Anwa*
Common: Cam wood

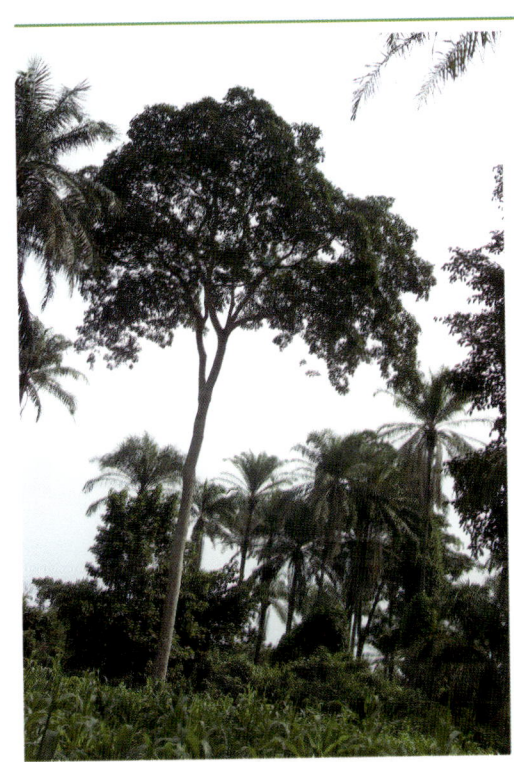

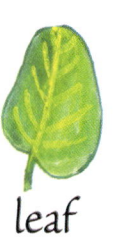

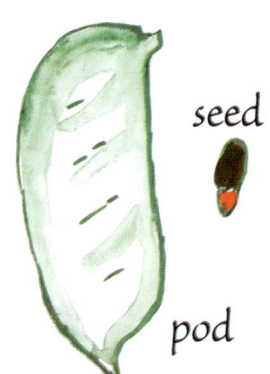

Family: *Caesalpiniaceae*

Up to 100 ft high and found in drier parts of forest regions. Flowers are very fragrant and green in colour with white and reddish markings on the petals. Fruits and seeds are black except for orange tips on the seeds.

leaf

seed

pod

•Medicinal

Good for treating headaches. Add some leaves to *ajaja* leaves and squeeze them; apply the liquid on to your forehead after making slight slits on the surface. Pain subsides immediately.

To cure malaria fever and jaundice the bark is soaked in cold water in which the sufferer bathes each morning until the sickness goes.

To treat skin diseases, *anwa, ogwujęba, ogichi* and *ajaja* leaves are ground to a paste with some water and applied to the affected area twice daily for 7 days. If severe, the affected part is washed with local soap before applying the paste.

This same formulation can also cure skin diseases in goats with engine oil used as a substitute for water.

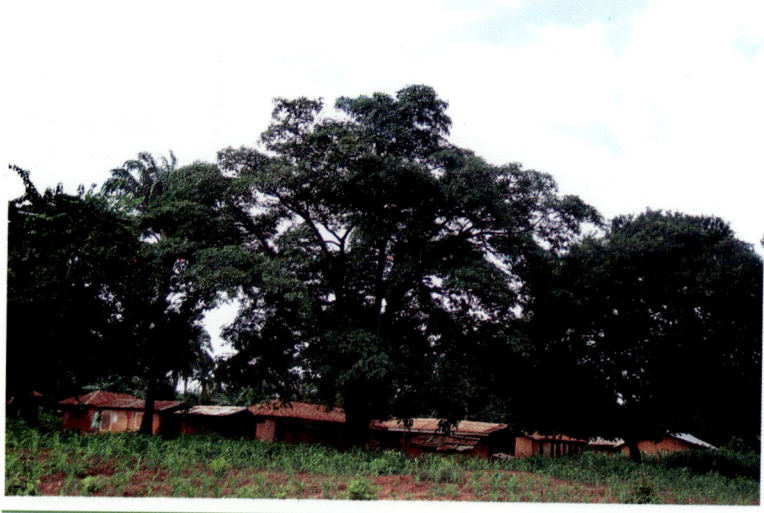

•Other uses

Anwa has long been prized as a firewood, but since it is now scarce and endangered it is no longer commonly used.

It provides an abundance of biomass all year.

Welcome shade in abundance in compounds and farms. Farmers store their yams (a highly valued crop) beneath it. A village (*Ofe-Anwa*) is named after it, thanks to an appreciation of its highly valued shade.

- Food

Its seeds are used for making soup.

- Cultural

This tree plays a pivotal role in Igala rituals. The pods are strung together with a string of old coins that have holes in the centre; the two ends of the string are joined to form a chain. The priests, as part of the ritual, throw the chain onto a carpet made of animal skin and invoke the ancestors.

The purpose of the consultation is to elicit from the ancestors what the future holds for them (fortune telling). There is a reluctance to accept monetary payment for such services as it makes the oracle unreliable.

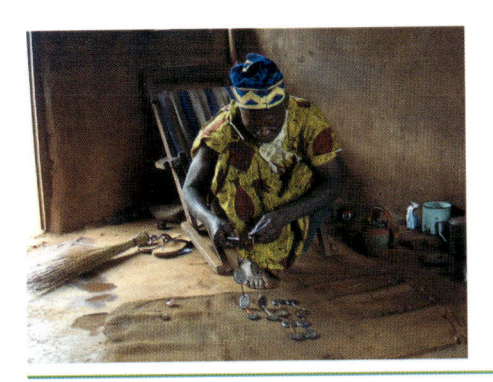

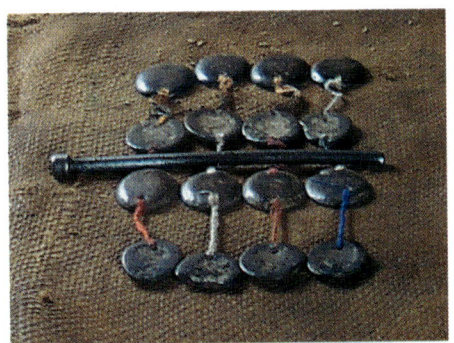

Local healers hold the same belief regarding payment.

Fortunetellers who are not priests also use these dried pods for the same ritual when consulting their oracle.

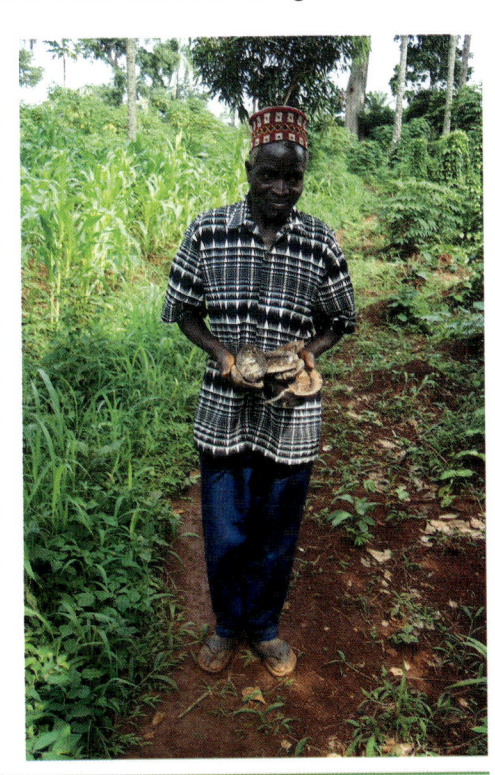

The difference between priests and fortunetellers is that in most cases priests take care of the idols; they regularly give them food and drink. Fortunetellers confine themselves to foretelling the future without the assistance of their ancestors.

The oracle looks like a statue and is the mediator between ancestors and priests.

The same pod when placed on top of valuable goods acts as a deterrent for thieves. Bad luck is in store for you if you steal any valuable goods covered with these pods.

It is believed that it will attack the descendent of the thief by cutting its mouth. To help differentiate a thief from the proprietor, the latter can harvest the crop safely provided they wear the same clothes that they wore initially. If not the mouths of future generations - children and grandchildren - will be damaged before birth.
Ẹbo onua kiya kimọtọ aluda

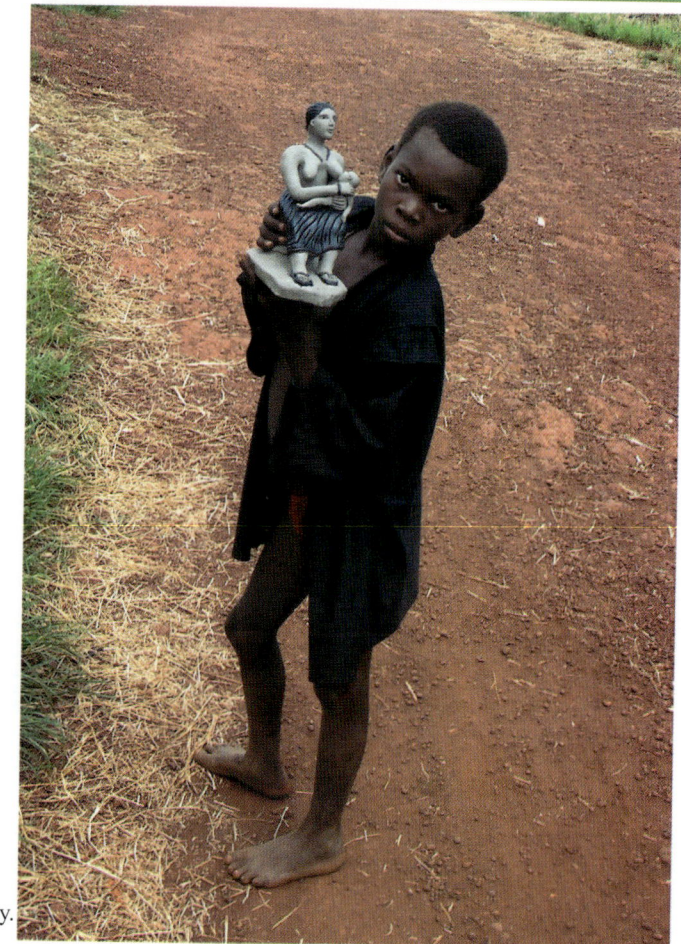

Picture shows a child holding an idol made of clay.

•Other uses

Anwa is recognized as the best plank for tables, beds, chairs, cupboards and doors. Its planed wood is beautiful, especially when stained with varnish which emphasizes its grain.

However, it is susceptible to woodworm. Despite this, it has become the most expensive wood in the market and now preferred to *iroko*, a tree of high renown on the African continent.

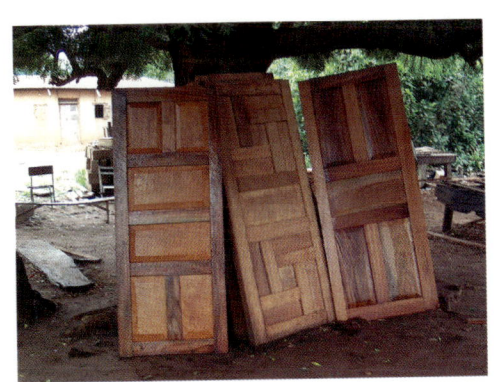

The fork stick of *Anwa* is used for local kitchens and parlours (*atakpas*).

It is also prized for roofing and granaries, and coveted for the construction of local houses where mud is plastered onto a frame of this wood (clay and wattle).

The seed is expensive, and Nigerian companies (particularly those involved in the cashew trade) buy it for export. The wood forms part of the local export trade.

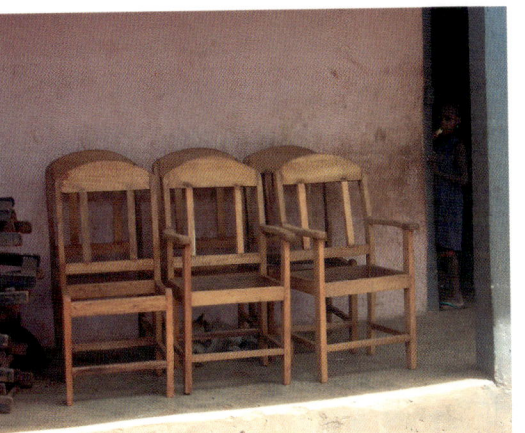

However, as lucrative as this resource is, Igalas are reluctant to invest in its production as it takes 7-8 years from planting to harvesting.

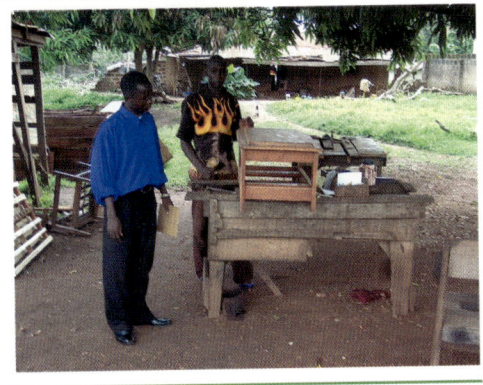

Annacardium occidentale

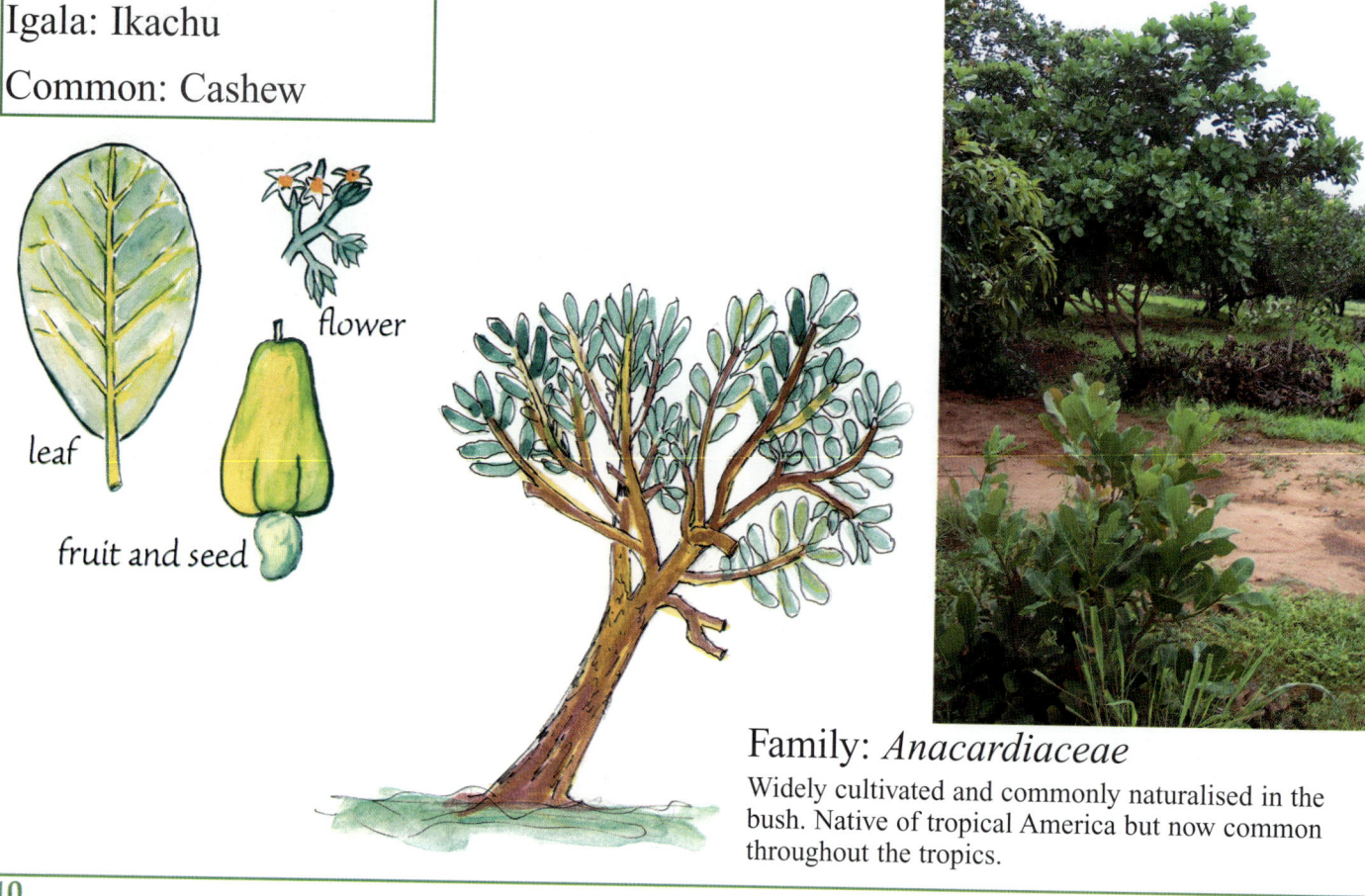

Igala: Ikachu

Common: Cashew

leaf

flower

fruit and seed

Family: *Anacardiaceae*

Widely cultivated and commonly naturalised in the bush. Native of tropical America but now common throughout the tropics.

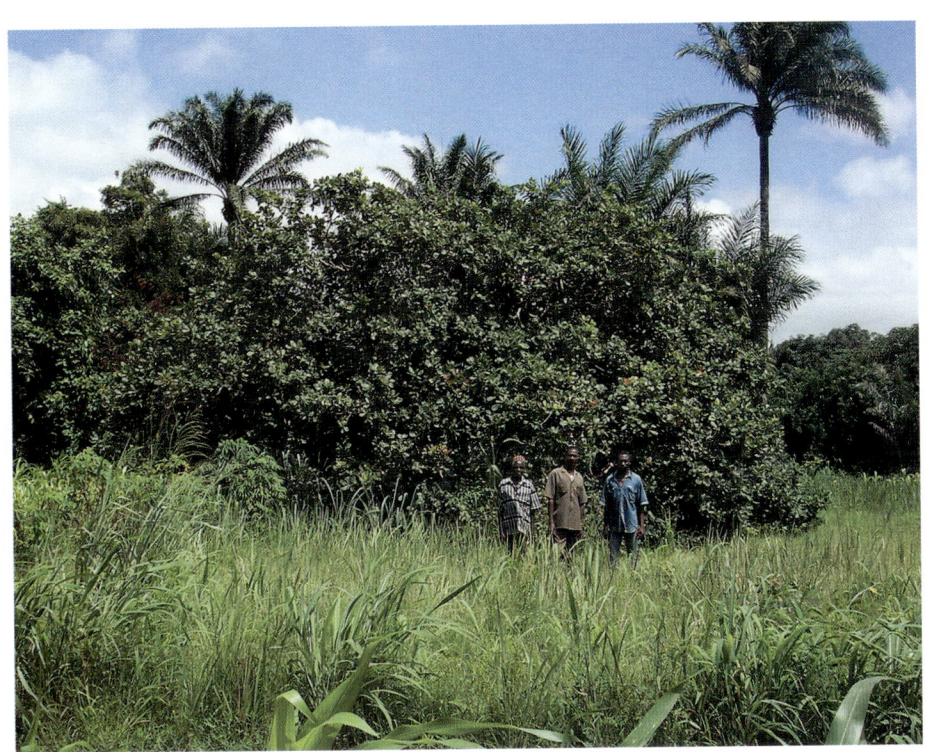

•Food

The fruit and nut are good supplements to all diets. Its juice is now becoming popular as a drink.

A sophisticated roasting process, known to most children, is used to extract the nut.

The skin bursts to release the nut which is then stored in an airtight bottle often sold along the highway. Eaten as a snack, it is now highly acceptable, with a market value higher than peanuts.

However, it is unfortunate that more cannot be done to guarantee better income for the producers as it has a high export value.

•Cultural

Planted along boundaries to delineate plots as well as providing boundaries for newly acquired land.

Children use its juice to tattoo their skin, writing their names on their hands.

•Medicinal

This tree derives popularity with those who fall victim to one of the commonest and most debilitating diseases in Igalaland, namely typhoid fever. Its fresh leaves are added to leaves of the umbrella tree (African almond), partially dried mango leaves, guava and eucalyptus leaves. The leaves are covered with water and boiled. The dosage is 1 glass, heated, 3 times daily for 7 days.

If typhoid is severe add a malt drink (such as Maltex) to the above mixture. An alternative method is to soak the cashew leaves, then squeeze them and add the liquid to a malt drink. The dosage is the same.

To treat scabies (*jẹdi jẹdi*), dysentery and malaria, combine and boil fresh and tender cashew leaves with guava, mango, banana and *Ijili* leaves. The dosage is half to one glass (infant or adult) 3 times daily for 7 days. It is first warmed.

In case of scabies wash the affected area with the medicine, and if severe wash with local soap, before application.

Roofs must be kept clear of its branches because their acidic content can quickly cause damage.

•Other uses

While good for firewood it is not used much because of its economic value. Traditional seats which are made from it are passed from one generation to the next. Occasionally used to make *atakpas* (local parlours) but now so valuable as a cash crop that people choose alternatives. It makes good handles for hoes, cutlasses and axes. Children make catapults from it.

It is not suitable for biomass due to its acidic nature

As a shade tree it generally does not do well because its branches are too low - they even touch the ground in many cases. But there are some exceptions as can be seen in the picture below.

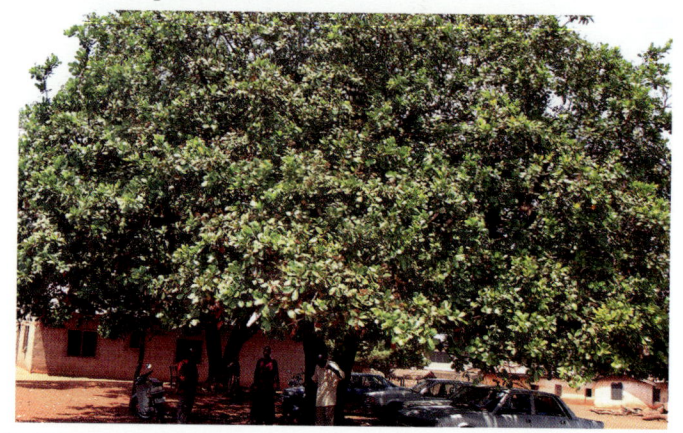

Anthocleista nobilis

Igala: *Odogwu, Odologwu*

Common: Cabbage Tree

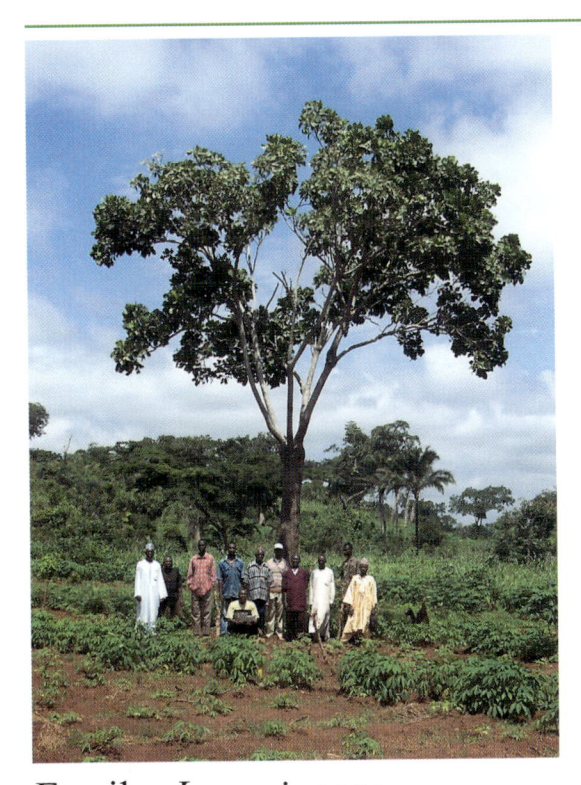

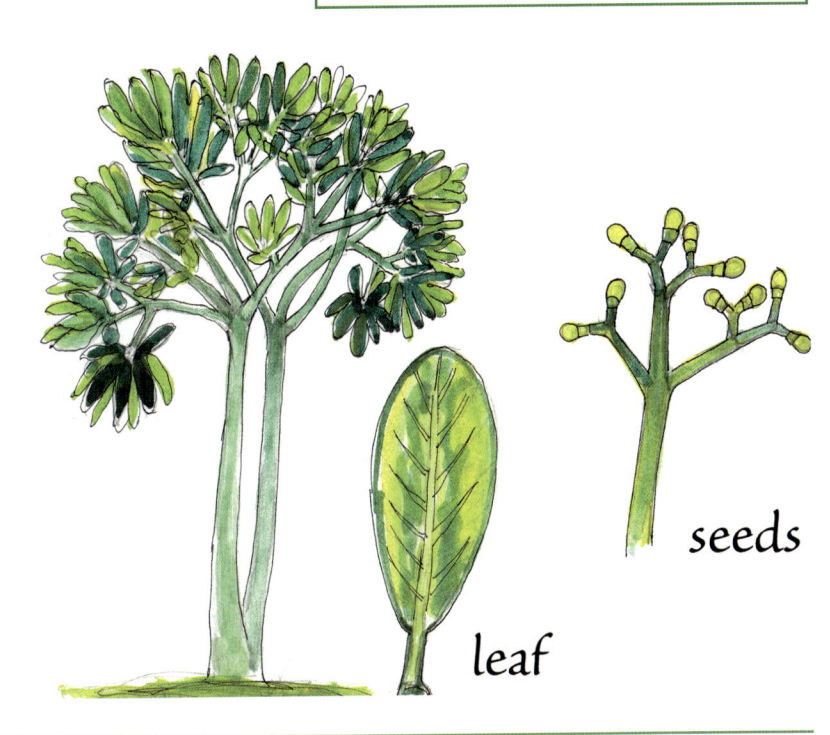

Family: *Loganiaceae*

25 to 60 ft high with a spiny stem and white flowers

leaf

seeds

•Food

Its seed is highly valued as a source of vegetable oil and vies with palm oil as a popular cooking oil, generating some local income.

•Cultural

Artists use it to carve images for traditional worship.

Ura (or Olubo) odogwu chunyi olulẹ ama, olule ofe odugwu alukokogbe

The healthy shade of an odogwu is a good shelter for crickets, but crickets found under the shade of an odogwu are not good to eat as they have a bitter taste.

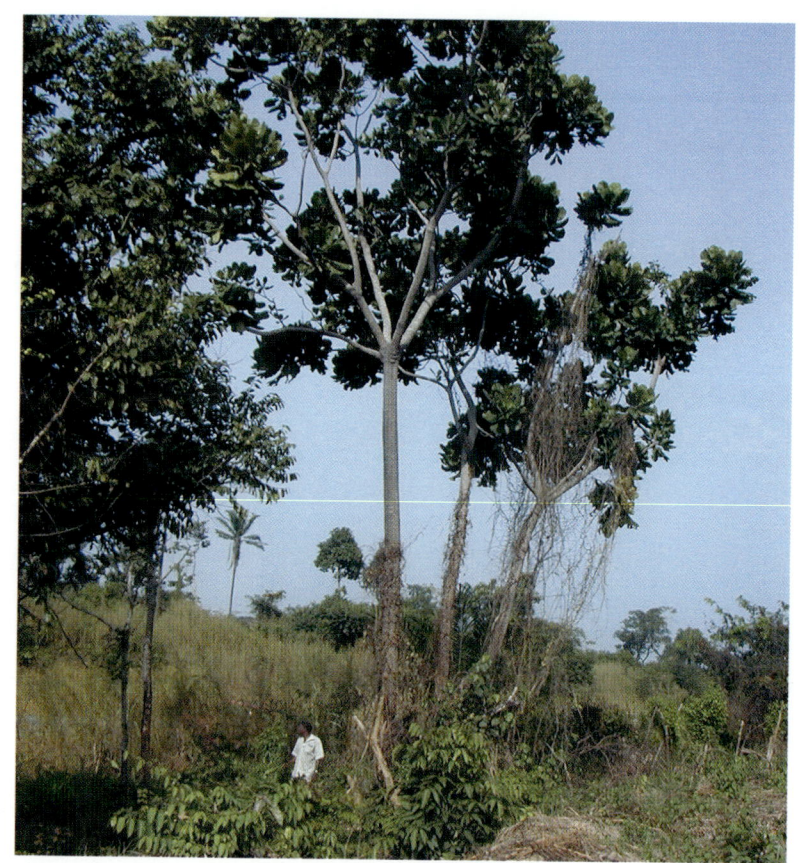

•Medicinal

It acts as a laxative, one of the symptoms of typhoid. The root is mainly used for the treatment of typhoid, dysentery and constipation. It is boiled with *otochi* and *Igbegbe* bark and *oyi* leaves. The dosage is 1 glass 3 times daily for 7 days. For more serious cases *otokwochi* leaves are added. It must be taken after food, otherwise it causes diarrhoea; only small doses are recommended because over dosage can also cause diarrhoea. For dysentery too it must be taken only in small doses.

To treat sexually transmitted diseases (STDs), the root is again used in combination with the leaves of *oyi* and *otokwochi*. The combined ingredients are boiled and taken while warm. The dosage is 1 glass 3 times daily for 5 months depending on the intensity of the problem.

If stomach ache has been caused by infection, eating different food or typhoid, the root is boiled with *oyi* leaves and the medicine taken while still warm. The dosage is 1 glass 3 times daily for 7 days. For persistent cases add *Ogele* and *ebe* leaves and *obulu* bark.

Health warning: only the female root can be used because the male root causes stomach ache. Experienced herbalists can distinguish between the two.

•Other Uses

It is not used much for firewood as the smoke causes dizziness. Traditional seats carved from it are handed down from one generation to the next.

Wheel rims for locally made trucks (dog carts) are made from it as well as traditional games.

As it is a soft and pliable wood artists use it for carvings. Although not recommended for buildings it is commonly used for temporary culverts.

Its leaves are used to cover the iron trap often used by hunters to catch animals.

Leaves produce lots of biomass. *Awolowo* grass (*Eupatorium odoratum*) grows well underneath it, providing evidence of fertility and moisture retention, although it does have acidic properties.

In riverine areas it needs to be supported by fork sticks, otherwise it falls on the ground, and is therefore not generally useful as shade. However, as the earlier picture shows, in upland areas its shade is much appreciated.

Some breeds of goat from the northern part of Nigeria eat its leaves.

Aubrevillea kerstingii

Igala: *Udu*

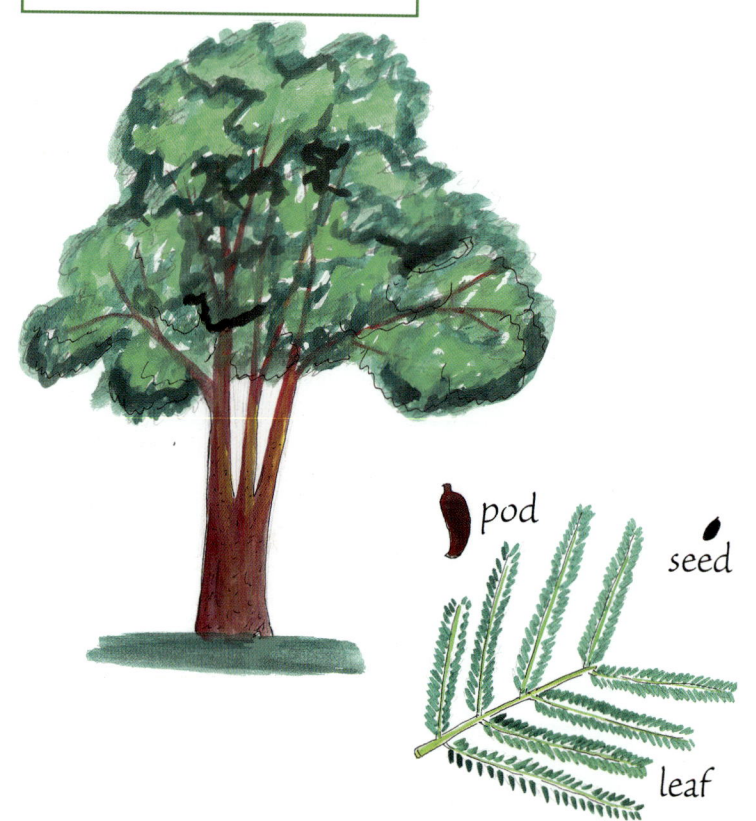

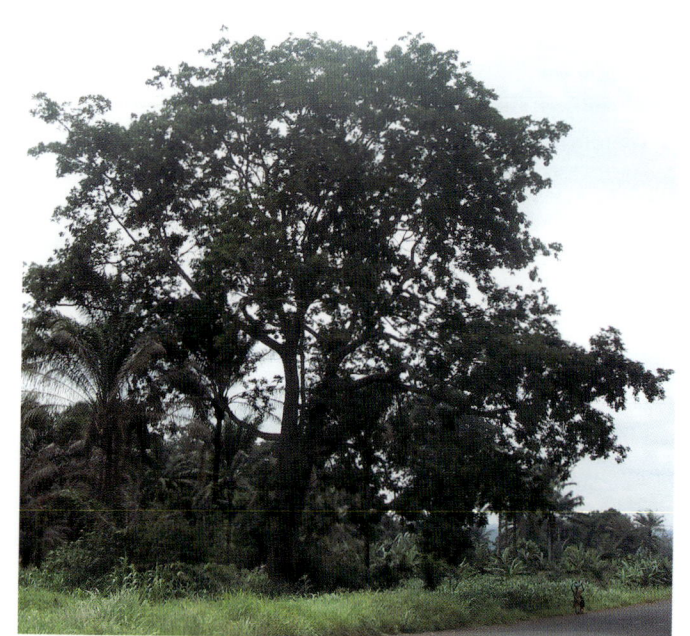

pod

seed

leaf

Family: *Mimosaceae*

Large forest tree growing up to 120 ft high. Has large buttresses and a spreading crown.

- **Food**

Udu fruits and leaves are edible and used for vegetable soup.

- **Cultural**

In olden days the *Udu* tree was the traditional place of sacrifice. The citizenry at large held that ancestors and devils cohabited beneath its shade. Traditionalists still believe this but Christians and Muslims tend not to.

It is believed that bush babies like the fruits, and children are advised not to go under it at night in case they encounter them

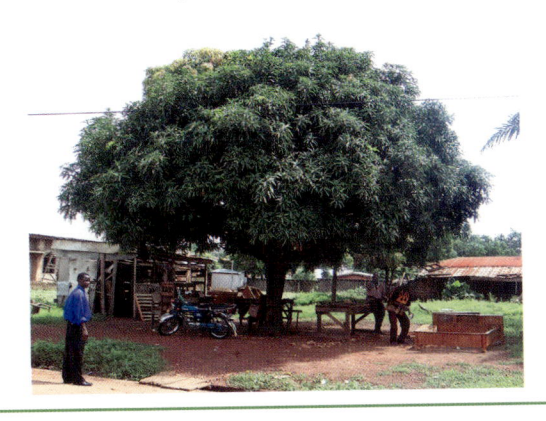

- **Medicinal**

The sap from its roots and leaves are used for stomach disorder (constipation) and worms.

It is also used for lower back pain, malaria fever and dysentery.

- **Other Uses**

It has an assortment of local uses and makes excellent planks for domestic and office furniture. As a hard wood not susceptible to woodworm, is ideal for morticing. Its timber is therefore expensive.

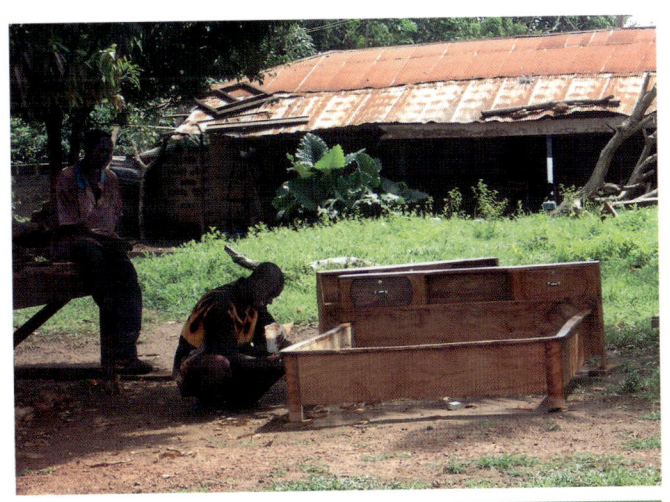

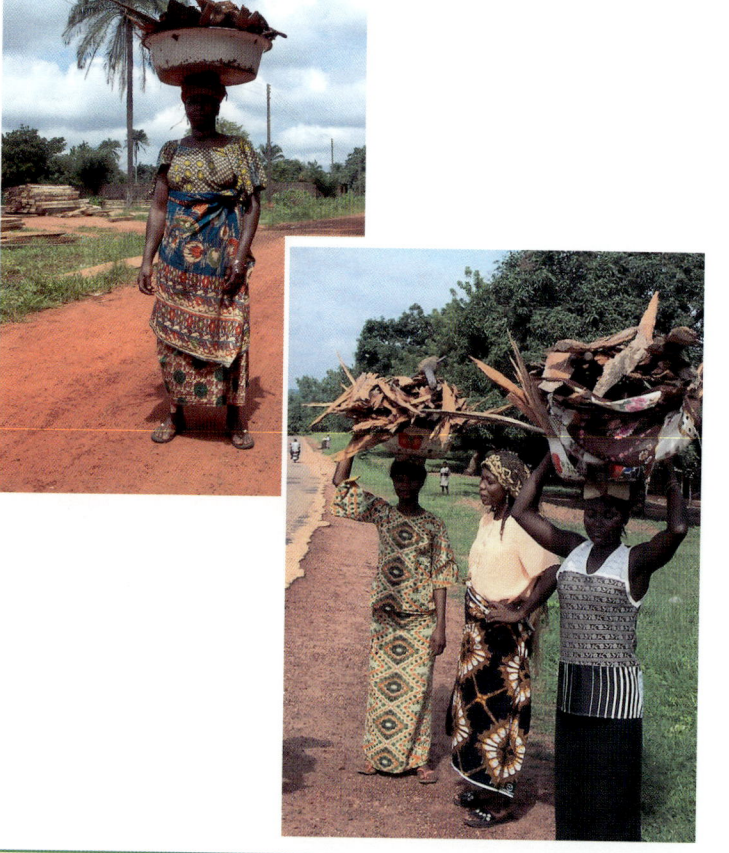

A highly suitable hardwood but, as an endangered species, is rarely used for firewood except in the north of Igala and south of Ankpa.

The women in the photograph have managed to obtain an old *udu* tree for firewood.

Fork sticks and branches are used for local building, granaries, animal stalls and staking of yams. Farmers hire casual labour to cut its fork sticks and branches. Ladders are made from it due to its durability, and fishermen use it for canoes.

Used for making the popular local games equipment (*ichẹ*), it is also crafted into mortars and pestles, handles for axes, hoes, cutlasses, catapults and the wooden part of Dane guns.

Udu has a superabundance of shade all year round which provides a good environment for women doing palm processing. Goats eat the leaves but in the process can destroy the tree.

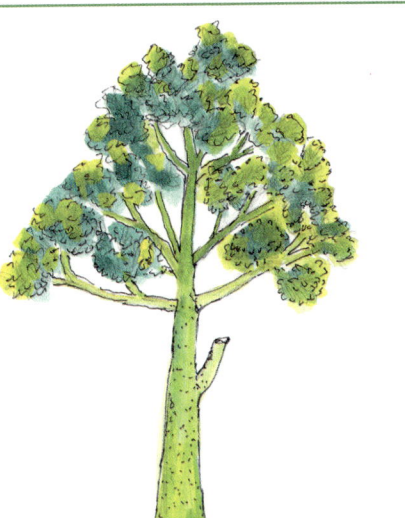

Azadiracta indica
Igala: *Oli-Ọda*
Common: Neem

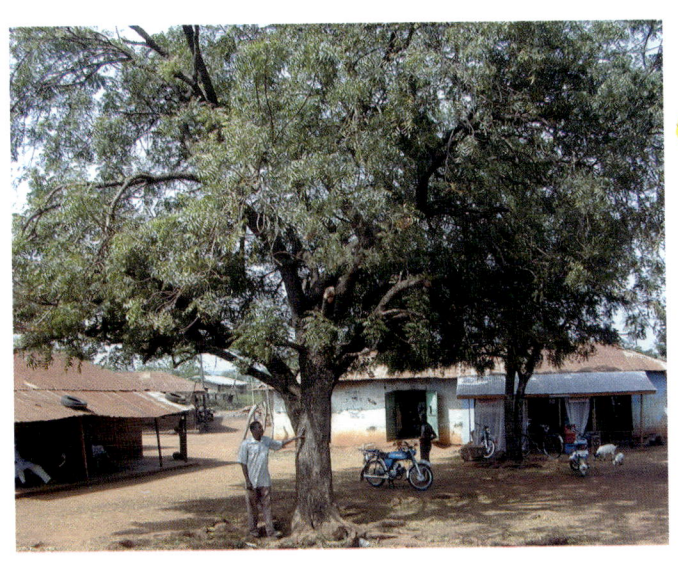

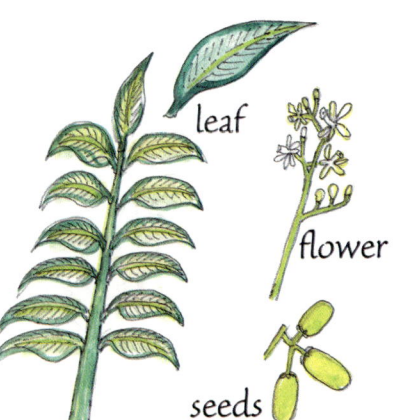

Family: *Meliaceae*

Evergreen tree up to 80 ft tall with abundant white flowers and yellow fruits. Native of India but now widespread throughout tropical and subtropical regions.

leaf

flower

seeds

19

•Food

The fruit and seed are edible but not commonly eaten. This is surprising given the sweetness of the fruit. However, people are generally wary of eating fruits.

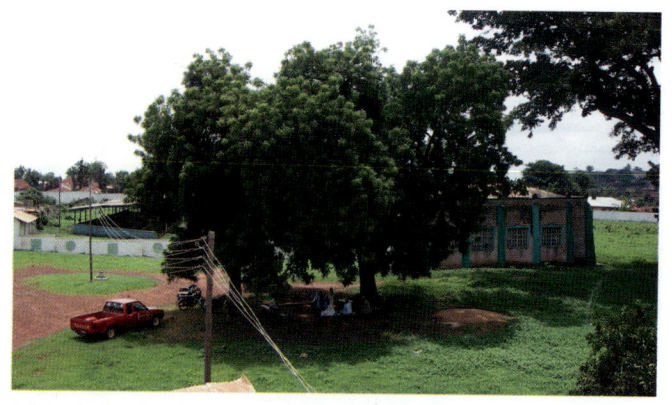

Neem tree in the grounds of the Attah of Igala's palace, Idah. Idah stadium is in the background.

•Cultural

It is used for boundary demarcation.

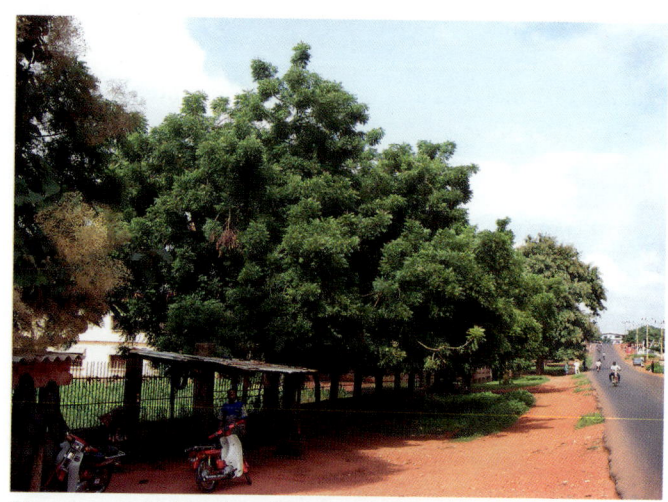

Use of neem for boundary demarcation along a road in Idah

As part of the Muslim burial rites, a layer of neem leaves is placed on top of the corpse after laying it in the grave (Moslems bury their dead without a coffin).

The grave is then filled and the neem protects the body from coming into contact with the soil.

•Medicinal

Neem enjoys high status in the world of traditional treatment. If the tree is in your compound you will have visitors on a regular basis all in need of various parts. A newcomer soon learns that the most common disease in Igalaland is malaria, and neem is a cure. The wood from the stem is put inside a bottle of local gin and soaked overnight. Dosage: 1 glass 3 times daily for 7 days. Many Igalas bear testimony of recovery from malaria fever resulting from leaves soaked in cold water and 1 glass taken 3 times daily for 7 days.

It also offers effective relief from toothache. For this you squeeze the leaves and soak them in cold water or gin (*ogogoro*). In either case you put the medicine in your mouth and hold it there for a few minutes.

Mothers greatly appreciate its medicine, especially for children's diseases which are often difficult to diagnose. Leaves are soaked overnight and afterwards cooked in warm water. The child is then bathed in this water twice a day. Igalas vouch for a high success rate of recovery using this simple practice.

•Other uses

Its wood is considered a good alternative to some of the endangered fuel wood species because of its fast growth allowing it to be harvested in the second or third year. It requires little maintenance.

However, a health warning needs to accompany this good news: its taproots are not strong and therefore falls easily, causing damage to roofs and buildings.

Neem is a hard wood suitable for building and furniture, mortars and pestles and rural implements such as hoe and cutlass handles.

Its leaves and seeds can be transformed into storage 'insecticide' that competes with commercial products. Much research is still needed before its full storage and insecticidal potential are fully realised.

Neem leaves can also be sun dried, ground and mixed with water to form a slurry with which yam seeds can be treated and dried. This acts as a protection against fungal diseases and possibly nematodes.

•Other uses

Neem provides good shade; birds are fond of the fruit. It also produces a chewing stick and tooth pick both of which have a good local monetary value. Women engage in their sale to augment income.

However, neem can easily become a weed.

Yet another hard wood suitable for furniture with many other uses, production is likely to increase in the near future.

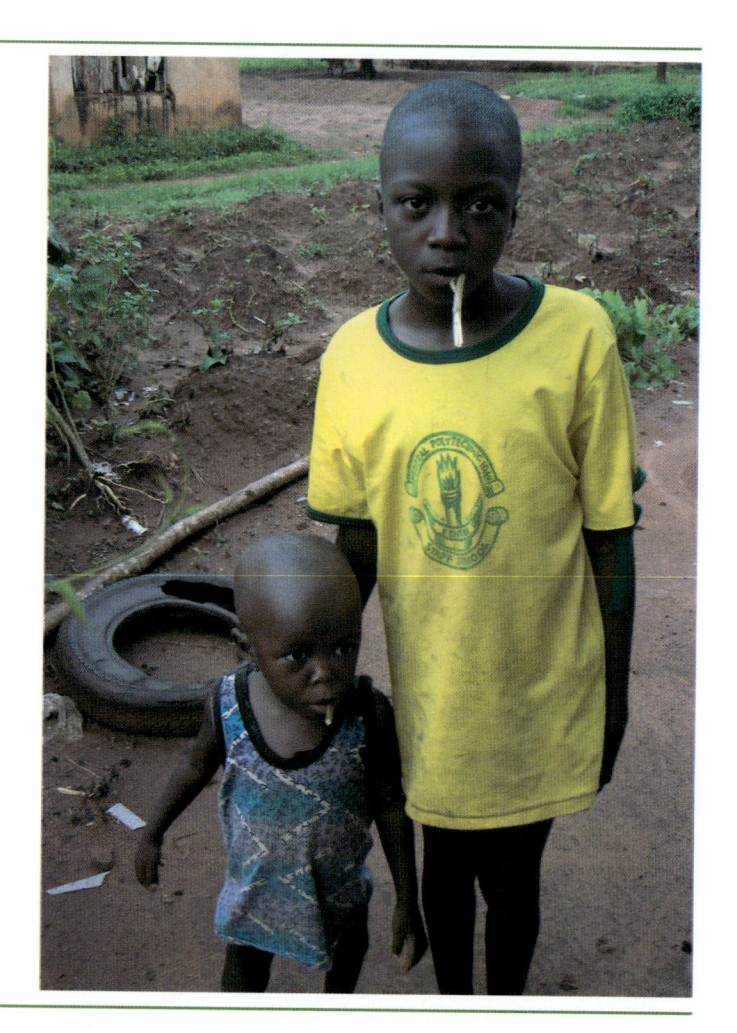

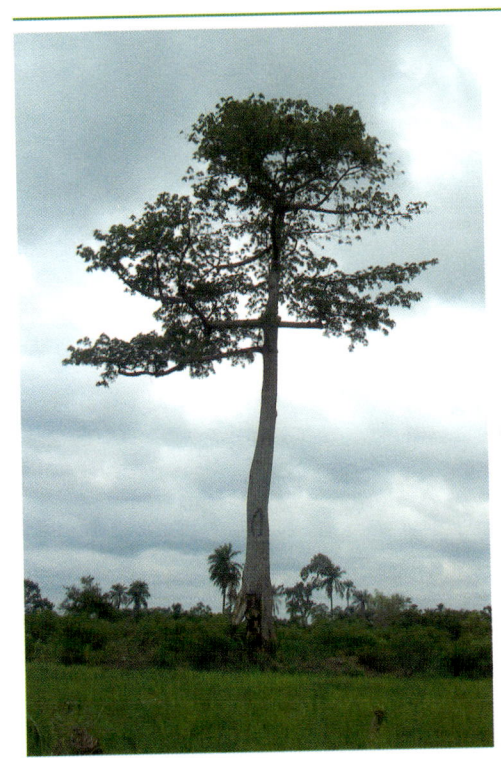

Bombax costatum
Igala: *Agwugwu, Agwu*
Common: Kapok tree

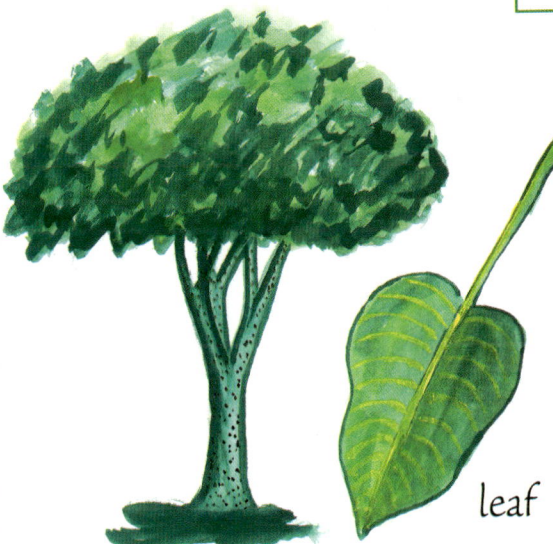

leaf

flower

fruit

seed

Family: *Bombacaceae*

Found in savannah regions, 10 to 50 ft high. Bark is usually rough and spiny. Flowers are red to orange in colour, sometimes yellow.

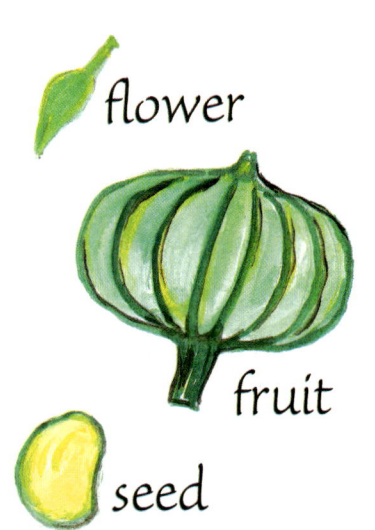

•Food

Fresh and tender leaves are used to make *draw* soup. Combining it with dried fish, salt, Magi (seasoning) and bitter leaf, housewives produce delicious *draw* soup in many parts of the region.

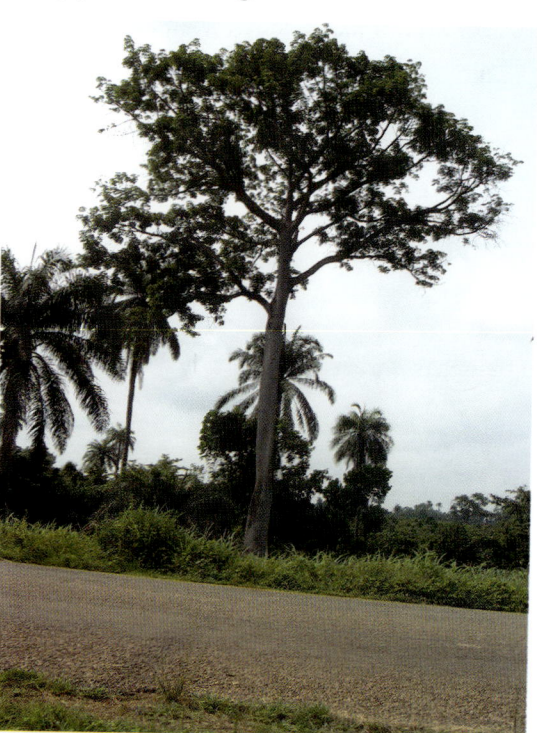

•Cultural

Local seats are carved from the trunk itself.

It ranks among those trees suitable for artifacts as well as other vital images of traditional worship. Statues for idols are carved from it as well as masks for local festivals.

Yet another popular tree for making local games (*ichi*) and durable drums.

So deep is its shade that it is possible to hide beneath it. For this reason it serves as a worshipping site and it is believed that bush babies (fairies) use it as their habitat. White and red cloth markings wrapped around its branches signify that it has been set aside as a place of worship. Fairies or bush babies are called *ichękpa*.

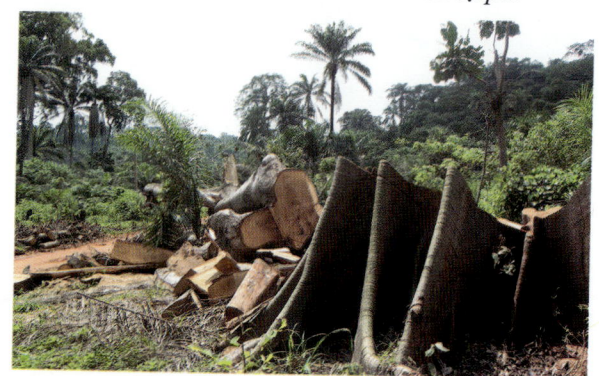

•Medicinal

There are two common species of Bombax, one smooth, the other thorny considered more suitable as food and medicinally important. Its leaves are used to relieve the pangs of child birth. Fresh leaves and bark are boiled; the drink is allowed to cool but re-heated before being administered. Dosage: 1 glass 3 times a day as long as needed.

To cure fever the bark is boiled with leaves of *ogele* and *alemu*. Dosage: 1 glass 3 times daily for 7 days after first bathing with some of the water.

To cure a peptic or stomach ulcer, the leaves are dried, then ground and prepared as okra soup. With the addition of bitter leaf, a popular Igala vegetable, it is eaten with corn food at least once a day until the ulcer is cured.

•Other uses

Regarded as a favourite fuelwood during the dry season. However, as a softwood it is unsuitable during the rains because it easily absorbs water.

Agwugwu is used for making office and domestic furniture, but considered to be inferior compared with *Afzelia africana* and iroko.

Boats, including canoes, are made from it though these are not used during the dry season which allows time for the wood to dry well. They can last up to 10 years if well maintained. The tree also produces a gum suitable for the repair of water craft.

Local seats made from it become part of the family heritage. If you cannot afford iroko you may resort to it for roofing. Handles for local knives, cutlass and harvesting tools such as diggers made from *Agwugwu* are coveted. Leaves and stems transform easily into biomass.

Bombax often has a layered structure like that of the umbrella tree. In the early stages of growth it provides shade but as it grows older the branches wither and fall. While young its foliage provides a safe haven for many a tired labourer, though the branches can sometimes be close to the ground. It therefore needs to be pruned for greater access to its refuge.

Goats can damage or even destroy the tree by feeding upon its leaves.

Local pillows and mattresses are often made from the fibres found in the pods.

Carica papaya

Igala: *Echibakpa*

Common: Pawpaw

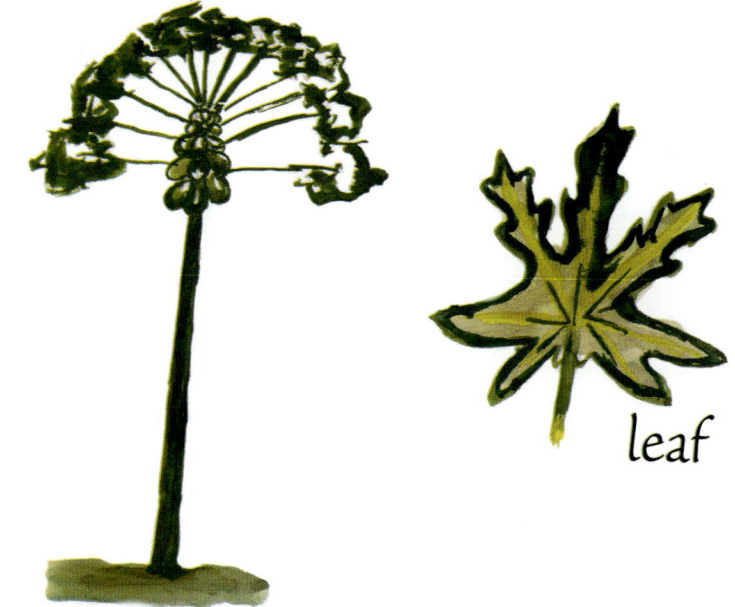

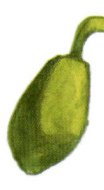

fruit

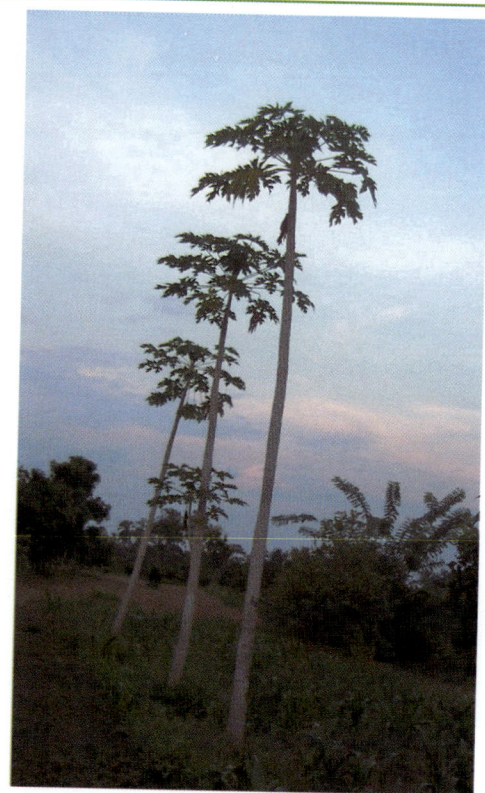

leaf

tree

Family: *Caricaceae*

A small family of plants mainly found in South America. Pawpaw is widely distributed and cultivated.

•Food

The fruit is popular as a snack especially among women who find it easy to prepare.

The unripe fruit can be sliced, boiled, mashed and served as a vegetable. The flavour of grated unripe fruit used for salad is improved by adding a little vinegar. Pawpaw is now commonly eaten; a change from 30 years ago when people were reluctant to try it.

Its literal meaning is Islamic Pumpkin (*Echi – Abakpa*).

•Cultural

Of no cultural value in the area.

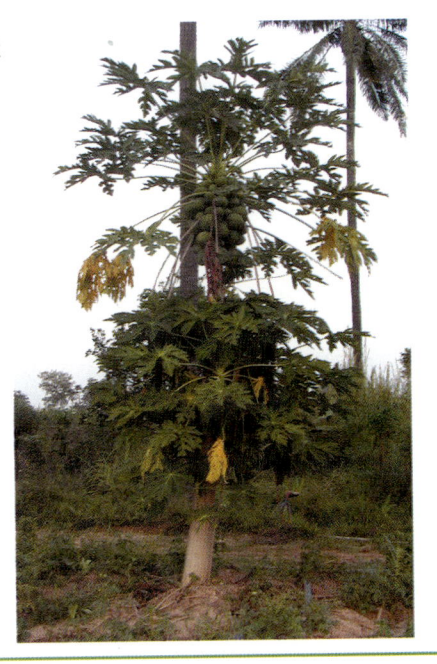

•Medicinal

Pawpaw is noted for its medicinal properties. By taking note of the type of leaves and parts of the tree a 'patient' is holding, one can tell the nature of the ailment.

Malaria fever is treated by the dry yellow leaves, which are boiled with avocado, mango and umbrella tree leaves. The dosage is a glass of this liquid 3 times a day for 7 days. The same drink cures typhoid fever.

If impotence is a problem, eat the whole fruit complete with skin, flesh and seeds once a day for 7 days.

To cure general aches and pains, pound the flesh of a ripe fruit to remove the juice. Mix the juice with Maltex (a malt drink) and take half a glass 3 times daily for 7 days.

Pawpaw, like Neem, is child friendly and children who suffer from convulsions are helped by it. Fresh leaves are combined with *ebe* and *ogẹlẹ* leaves and then boiled. The liquid is cooled slightly and then divided into portions for drinking and bathing. Give half a glass to the sick child, then bathe him/her in the remainder 3 times a day for 5 days.

To prevent malaria, eat the ripe fruit.

Unripe pawpaw fruit is used to cure peptic and stomach ulcers. Cut the unripe fruit into pieces and then soak in water with crushed garlic. Leave the mixture overnight. Dosage: 1 glass 3 times a day for as long as required.

A patient cured by this treatment reported that the mixture left to stand for 4-5 days fermented and turned to alcohol. The drink therefore must be made regularly.

Health warning: its dried leaves are more potent than Indian hemp and should not be consumed.

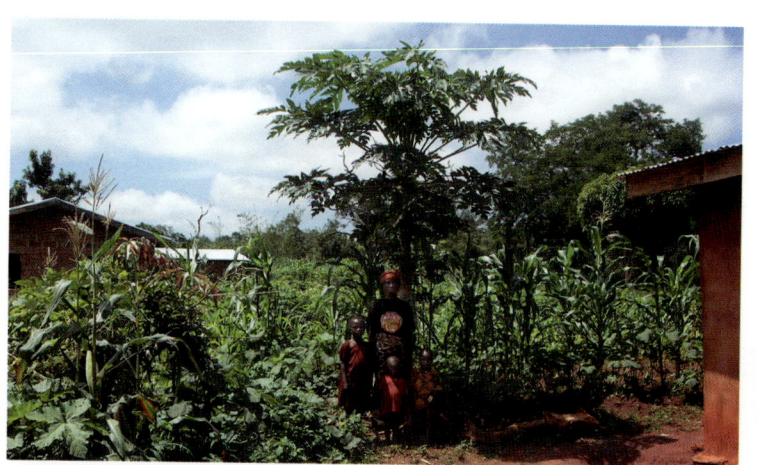

•Other uses

Because of its hollow trunk pawpaw is unsuitable for furniture. However, children use it to construct local trucks as a first step in mechanical engineering. They also make whistles from its leaves.

The leaves constantly fall to the ground giving good biomass as they decay easily. The stem also decays quickly and can be used for mulch or compost.

Animals eat the fruit that falls to the ground. Cattle usually like its leaves at all stages.

The fruits fetch a good price in the market because they are now regarded an important part of the diet.

As part of the food business it can be sold as snacks either whole or cut into slices.

The tree propagates easily and bears fruit within a year or two, requiring little maintenance.

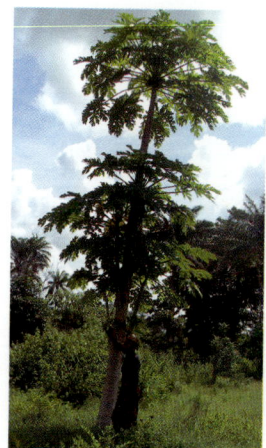

Chrysophyllum albidum
Igala: *Utẹ, Utiẹ, Ẹhia*
Common: African cherry

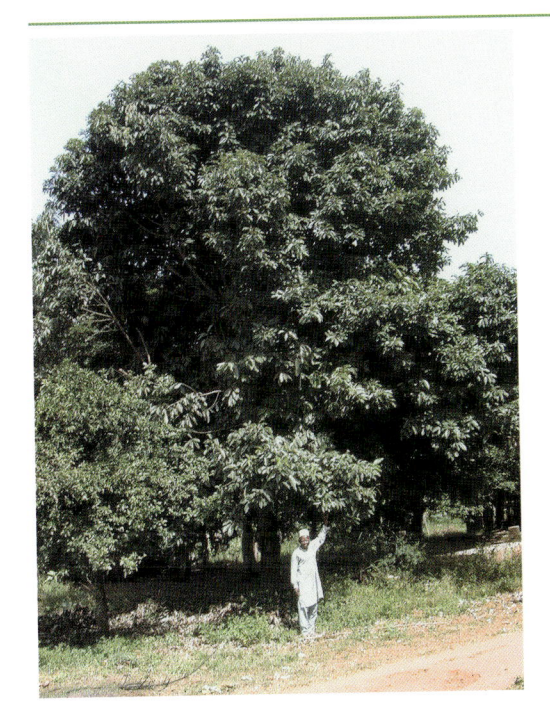

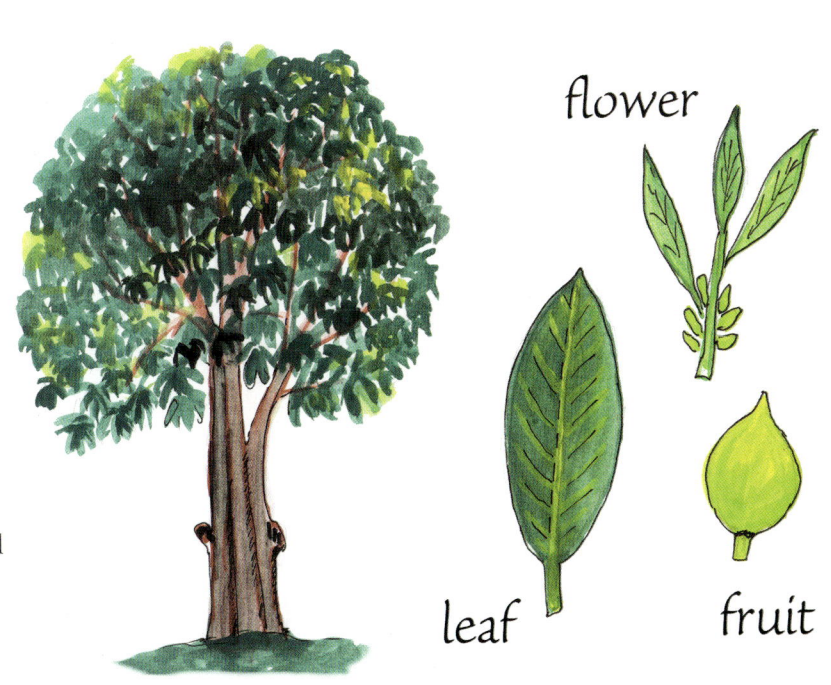

Family: *Sapotaceae*

Widespread in tropical Africa. Tall tree with small flowers amongst or below the upper leaves.

flower

leaf

fruit

•Food

The fruit is edible.

•Cultural

The seeds are dried and made into waist and ankle bands used in cultural dancing at festivals.

Under the African Cherry
bush babies and others are always found.
So anybody coming to collect the fruits must shout
to scare them away

Ene, ene, ene or Enooo or Ẹnẹdọmọ, Amo mamẹ,
amaooo...

•Medicinal

The leaves are cooked for pregnant women who are recommended to take the drink 3 times daily throughout the pregnancy.

It improves lactation for mothers who have little breast milk.

To cure obesity and oedema the bark is boiled and a glass of the liquid taken 3 times daily for 7 days. Women and men with these ailments are treated similarly.

An alternative way of curing any of these problems is by bathing in the liquid every morning.

This mixture is yet another option for the treatment of malaria.

- **Other uses**

Once popular as firewood but now only used when the tree dies due to the value of its fruit.

Much income is generated from its fruits, timber, seeds and firewood. It produces gum used locally but not yet commercially developed.

Domestic and office furniture can be produced from this hard wood, along with handles for axes, hoes and cutlasses.

The fork stick from prunings only is used for local buildings.

It gives excellent shade all year round and the leaves provide an abundance of biomass.

Goats eat the leaves and can damage the tree when young. Seedlings are normally fenced.

Its dark green leaves improve an otherwise monotonous landscape.

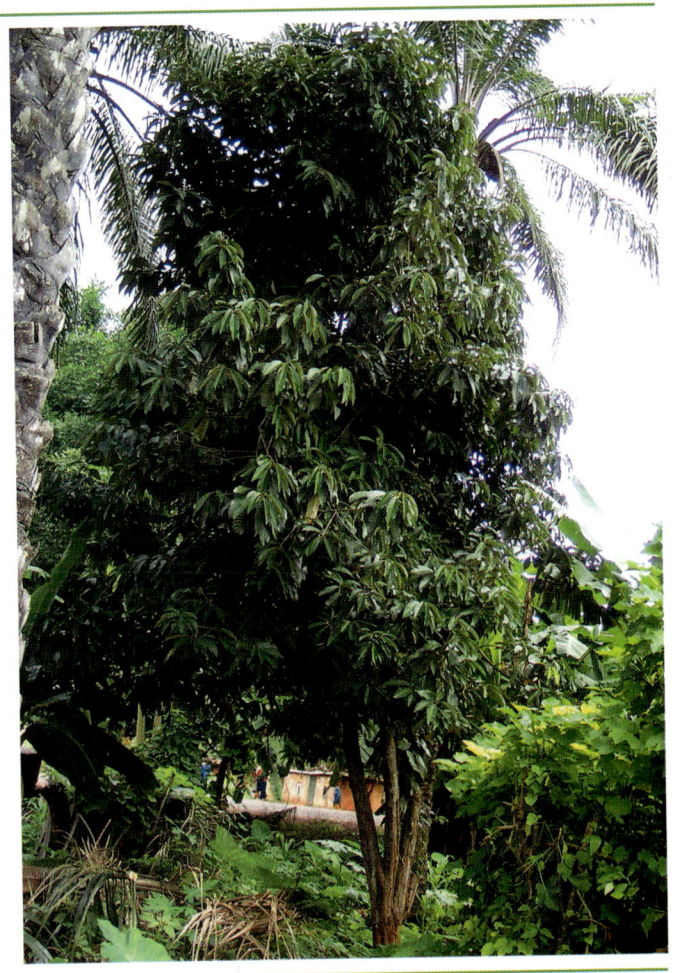

Citrus aurantium

Igala: *Alemu, Ulomu*

Common: Orange

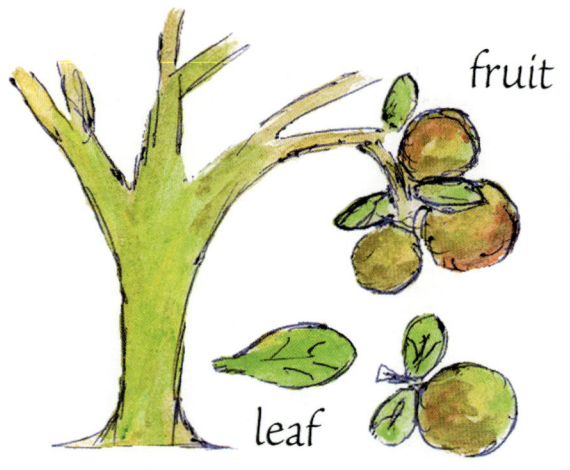

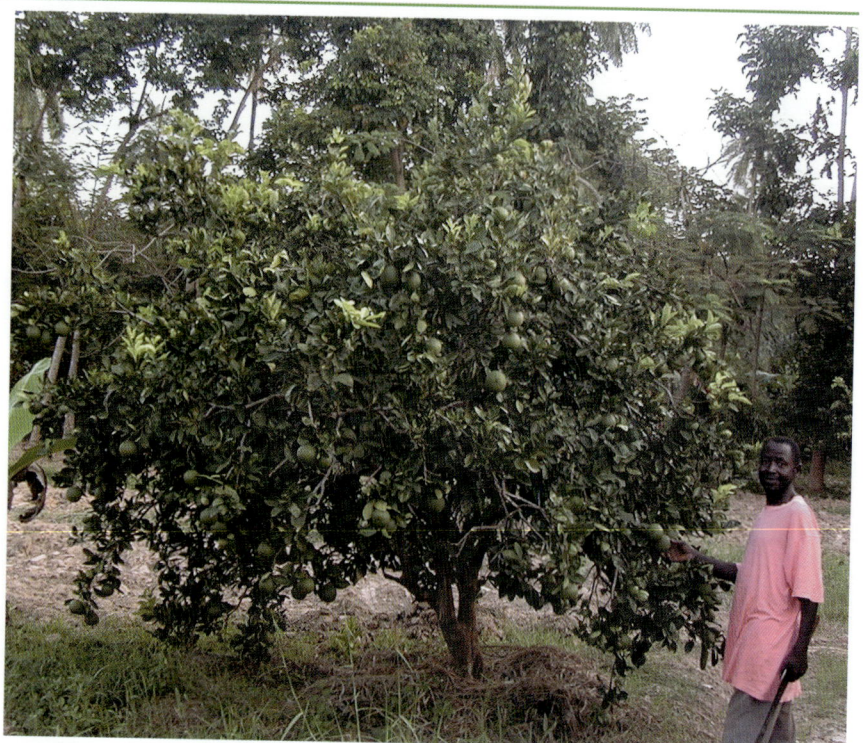

fruit

leaf

Family: *Rutaceae*

•Food

Oranges (sold green in the region) have become part of the diet especially when in season. They can be seen for sale in almost every market, and by the roadside.

Oranges are eaten in a hygienic manner with the outer skin shaved and the top sliced off. Everyone, even the smallest child, is adept at doing this. The cut end is placed in the mouth and the juice squeezed through. Oranges are not usually sectioned and eaten whole. The residue after drinking is excellent for composting.

Orange juice is recommended as part of the weaning food for babies given on a spoon, and as a good source of vitamins, particularly vitamin C.

Oranges are sold at good prices as demand far exceeds supply.

To market the oranges the owner sometimes sells the orange tree for a season to a trader. This makes it easy for the tree owner to derive revenue without worrying about the cost of labour at harvest time.

Dwarf varieties of orange are now being encouraged as these facilitate harvesting.

Orange trees can be very thorny.

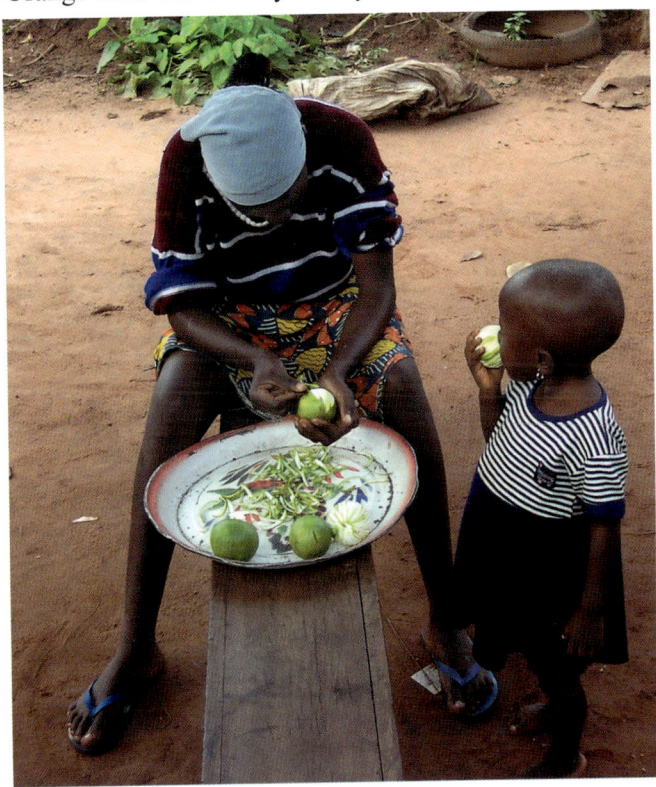

•Cultural

Oranges made their debut in this region during the latter half of the 20th century.

The Canadian Holy Ghost missionaries planted seedlings in every out-station they visited. This is particularly evident between Ankpa and Abejukoko where some of the orange trees are still to be found.

The first real citrus orchard was established by a Mr Lomax during the colonial period in Ayangba. Considering this and the virtual non-use of citrus previously, it is obvious that rapid progress has been made.

Like neem, orange sticks are also used for chewing.

•Other uses

Old trees are burned for firewood despite their thorns. Orange wood is not used for furniture or building because of the thorns, but can be utilised for hoe, axe and cutlass handles.

It provides a lot of shade, but the tree can harbour snakes. Don't walk under the tree at noontide!

Goats eat the flowers that fall from the trees and eat the peel and fruit if given the opportunity.

Nothing is more beautiful than an orchard in full white blossom, with the wonderful pervasive perfume it exudes as a bonus.

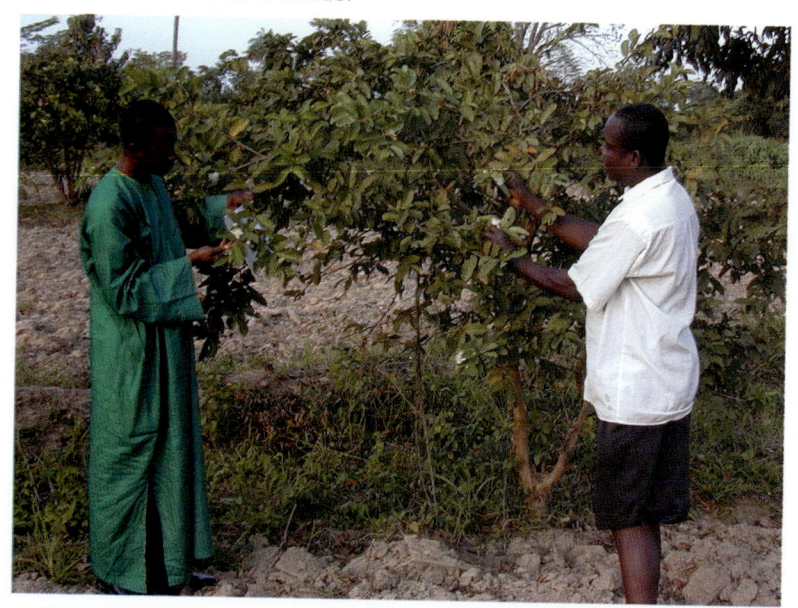

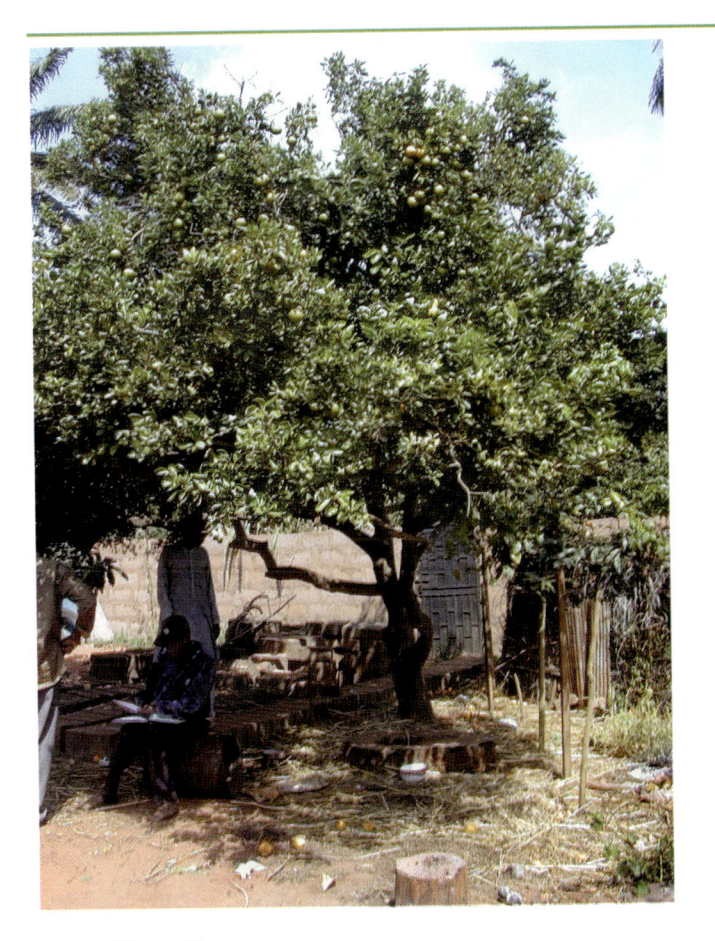

Citrus X tangelo
Igala: *Alemu-Itajalini*
Common: Tangerine

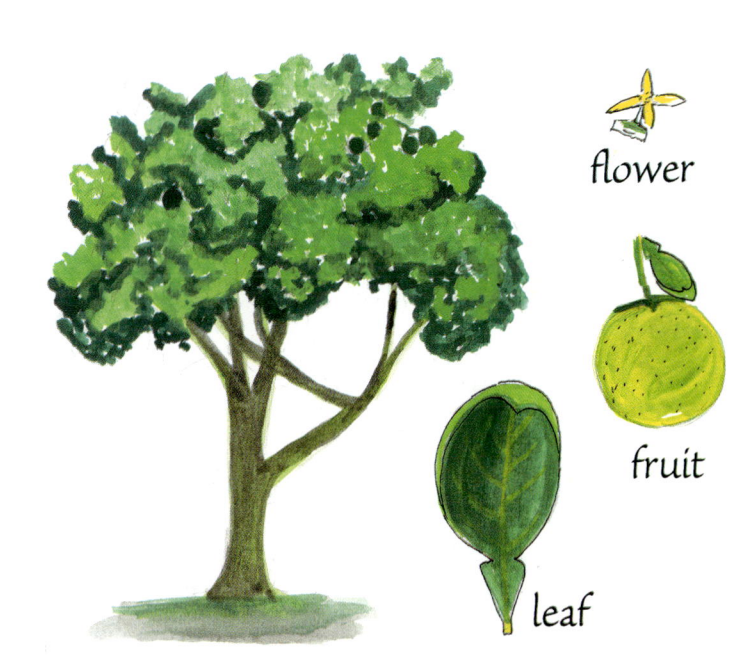

flower

fruit

leaf

Family: *Rutaceae*

A close cousin to the orange, the tangerine can equal whatever the orange provides and has great potential.

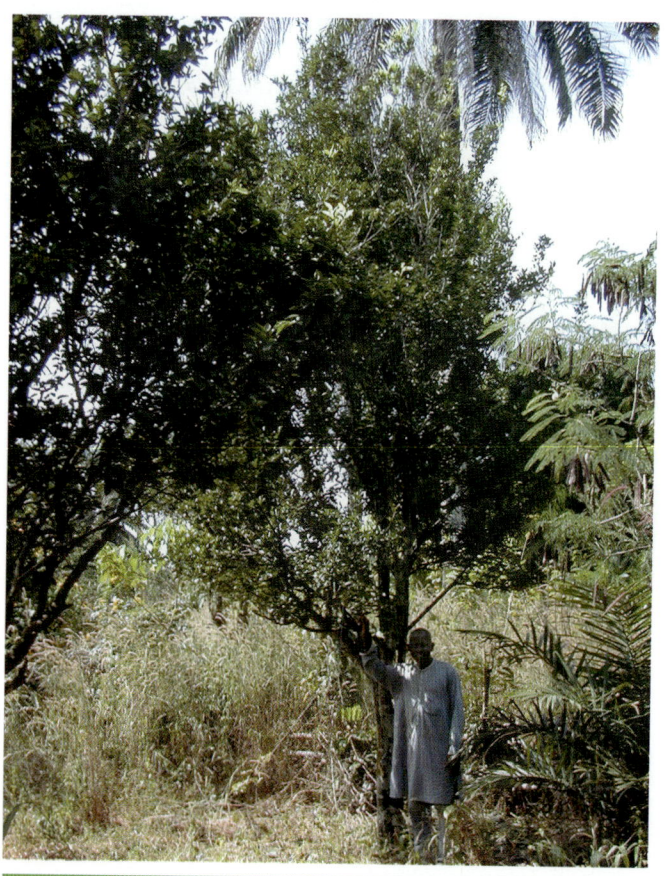

The fruit, though still new, has become widely accepted, as it is sweet and easy to peel. The tree takes 3 to 4 years to bear fruit. Most farmers cannot afford to wait this length of time as they need a quick return on their investment.

The tree is lower than the orange and its shade preferred.

Tangerines sell well but are still scarce in the market, some preferring them to oranges.

The tree looks prettier than the orange with fewer thorns and a smooth trunk.

Owners protect it from goats using forked sticks.

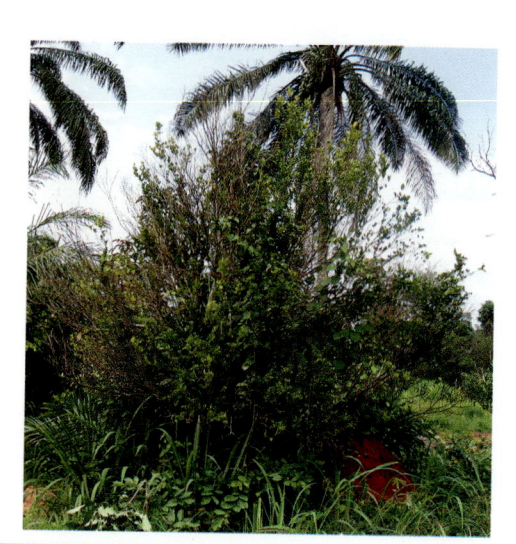

Cocos nucifera
Igala: *Unọba*
Common: Coconut

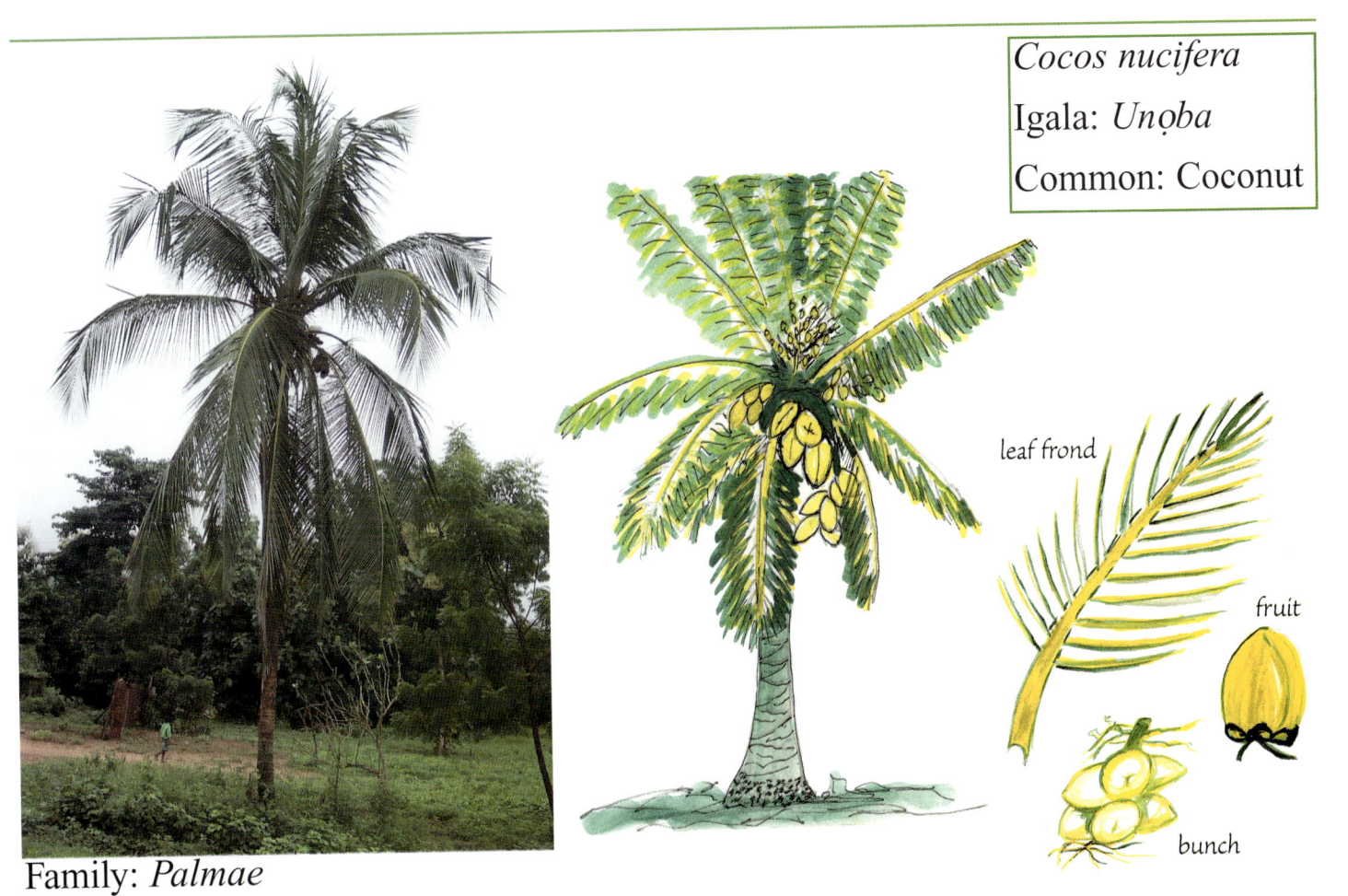

leaf frond

fruit

bunch

Family: *Palmae*

37

•Food

The latex (fluid inside the fruit) is consumed as a refreshing drink. Everyone relishes its white flesh taken as a snack or as an accompaniment to many dishes especially fresh roasted corn, *gari*, groundnut and garden egg. It is also eaten with dried cooked corn to enhance the flavour.

•Medicinal

The latex is drunk as an antidote to poison, alcohol and drug overdose. Drinking the latex also helps revive a person who has fainted or who has a reaction to an injection; it will also cure stomach ache in children.

The latex from a whole coconut when divided and taken morning and evening for 14 days will prevent goitre.

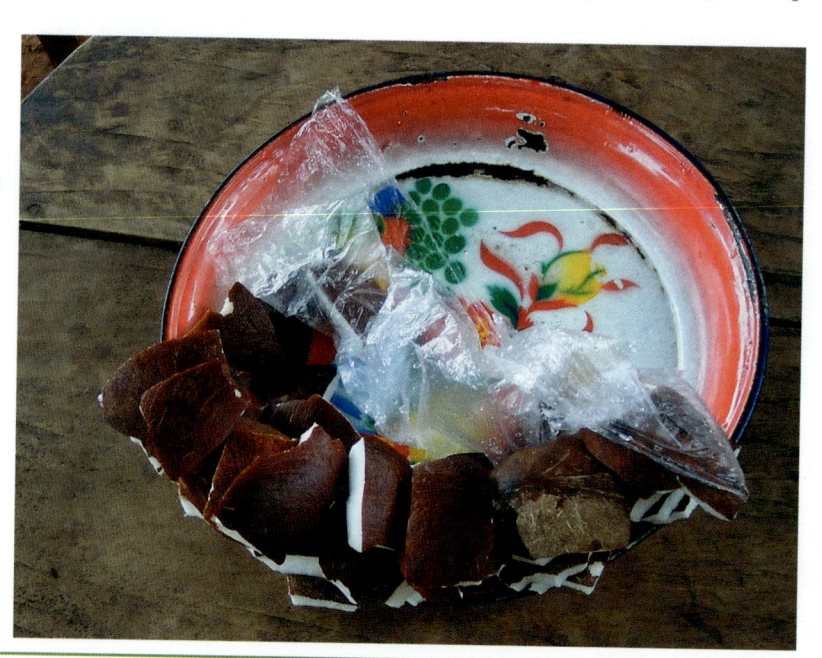

To cure eczema, rub the latex onto the skin. For a better result the latex can be mixed with sulphur.

Those with stammers rub their mouths with the coconut shell each morning, believing it helps them.

•Cultural

There is a belief that if you pour the water from the coconut on the heads of children it will increase their height, but it is also said that the liquid can create bad luck.

Local song:
Amalukomile kiwe fu-unoban

•Other uses

Its deadwood and fallen leaves serve as firewood.

It is not suitable for furniture, building, or tools, although brooms can be made from its leaves. Its shell when cut in halves is often used for polishing floors.

Hair Oil Food, the western label for women's hair oil, is made from coconut. Women soak the whole nut in cold water for 1 to 2 days after which they crack the mesocarp (middle shell) and pound the flesh. It is then used as hair oil - a real luxury providing excellent treatment for hair and scalp.

The tree provides good shade initially but often grows too tall to give much protection. The dwarf varieties are preferred as they are shadier and easier to harvest.

Goats feed on the leaves that fall to the ground.

By-products such as the hard fibrous casing are used for cleaning grinding stones.

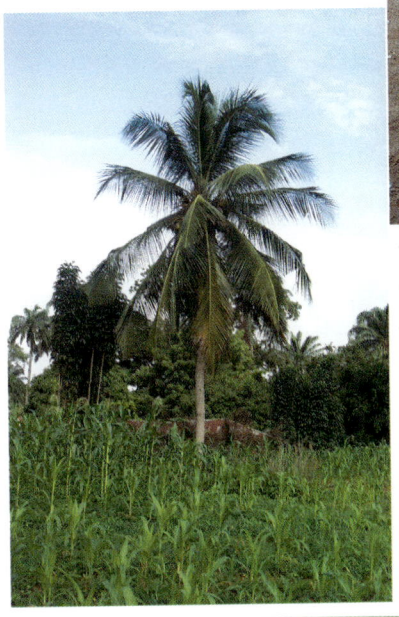

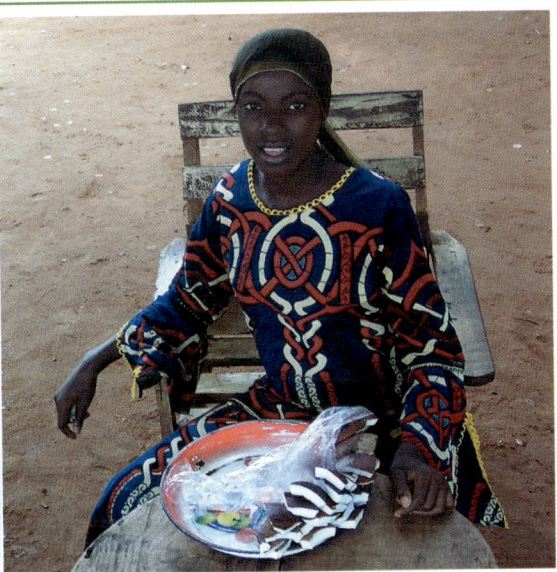

Selling pieces of coconut is a woman's way of supplementing income

Income-wise it is comparable to oil palm and an asset to families. It is much valued as a cash crop, especially by women.

They are sometimes planted as ornamentals to beautify the environment, and like the palm tree it too improves soil fertility. Note the green, healthy maize in the picture.

Cola acuminata

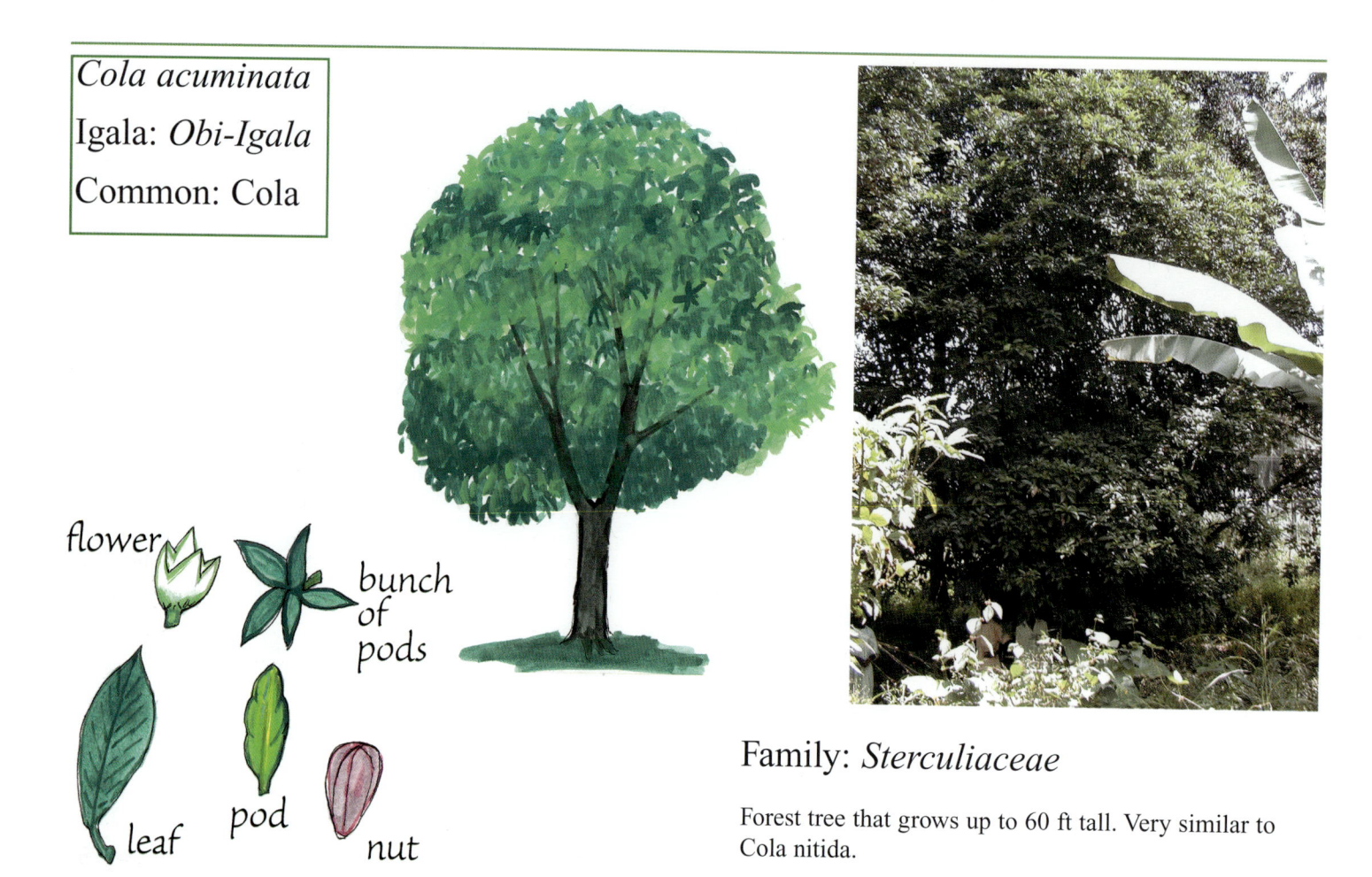

Igala: *Obi-Igala*

Common: Cola

flower

bunch of pods

leaf

pod

nut

Family: *Sterculiaceae*

Forest tree that grows up to 60 ft tall. Very similar to Cola nitida.

•Food

Obi-Igala has no value as food, but it is often chewed as a stimulant. *"Cola lasts in the mouth of those who value it,"* the saying goes.

"Obi akpọkpẹ ebulu abo kuma li ojinma."

•Medicinal

For the treatment of stomach ache, boil its leaves with *ebe* and *ọgẹlẹ* leaves. Dosage: 1 glass 3 times daily for 7 days.

•Cultural

The traditional symbol of hospitality in Igala and Bassa lands, cola is offered to all guests only after they have partaken of water.

Cola marks the tombs or graves where ancestors are laid to rest; a tribute paid only to chiefs, titleholders, traditional priests and elders.

When broken into pieces cola becomes an oracle used to consult the ancestors.

During traditional festivals the cola is offered to the ancestors as a mark of respect, as traditional believers understand they still need to feed their deceased forbearers.

Marriage ceremonies rely heavily on cola as entertainment at every stage from engagement to the marriage ceremony itself. Idol worshippers offer cola to their gods each time they perform sacrificial duties.

A suspect of a crime in a community must first provide cola for the community leaders of his/her own age grade before being judged by them. If found guilty of the offense cola is prescribed in the first stage of reconciliation.

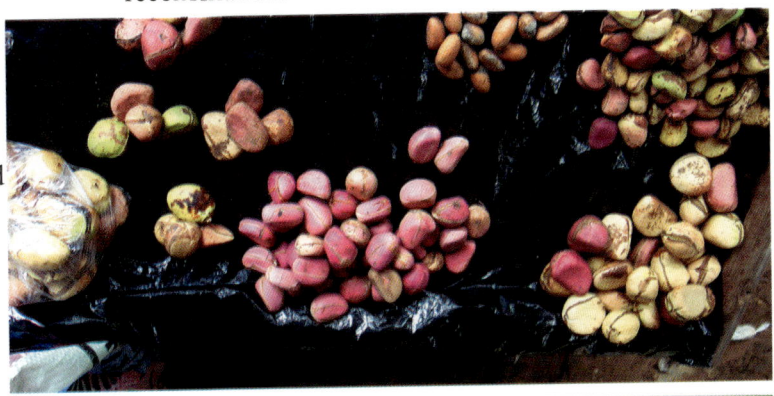

Traditional healers take cola from their patients as a sign of respect. In the ensuing ritual it is broken and shared with patient, healer and relatives who come with the patients.

Fishermen offer cola to the gods of the river before the commencement of the fishing season.

During land allocation cola is offered to the land owner before negotiations proceed.

No matter how small the colanut it still maintains its respect before the ancestors
Ekpana obi kimanya rajina.
If the nuts fall onto each other (cross themselves) it means that death will occur.
Ogbodaga ifa ibi kima nepi or Ogbodago akoia majabi

•Other uses

Because it rates among the top 10 cash crops in the region it is rarely used for firewood except when the tree dies. For the same reason it is no longer used for furniture.

Even though its fork stick would serve well in the construction of local dwelling houses, no one would be foolish enough to use it.

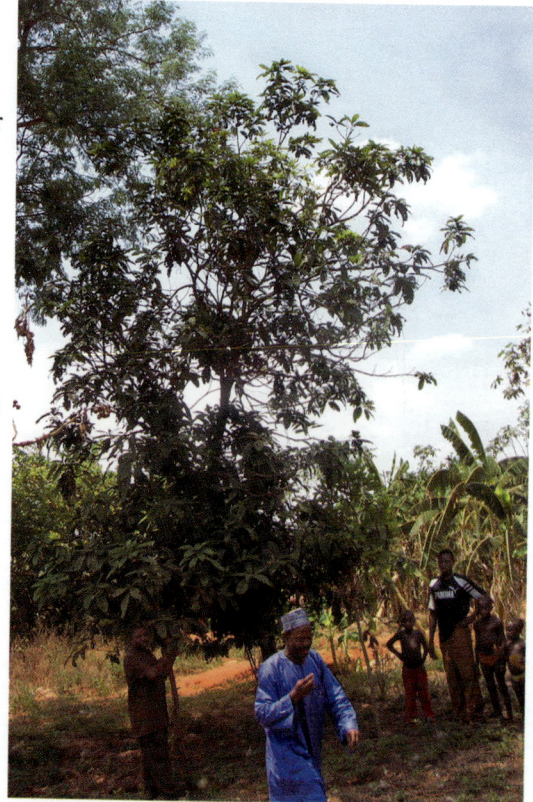

It fertilises the soil beneath and around it with an abundance of biomass. As it does not tolerate any form of maltreatment it is worthless as shade. Neither has it any value as fodder.

Its ornamental qualities enhances the region, especially during the rainy season when its leaves are dense.

Cola gigantea
Igala: *Ugo, Ebenebe*
Common: Cola

leaf

pod

pod (section)

seed

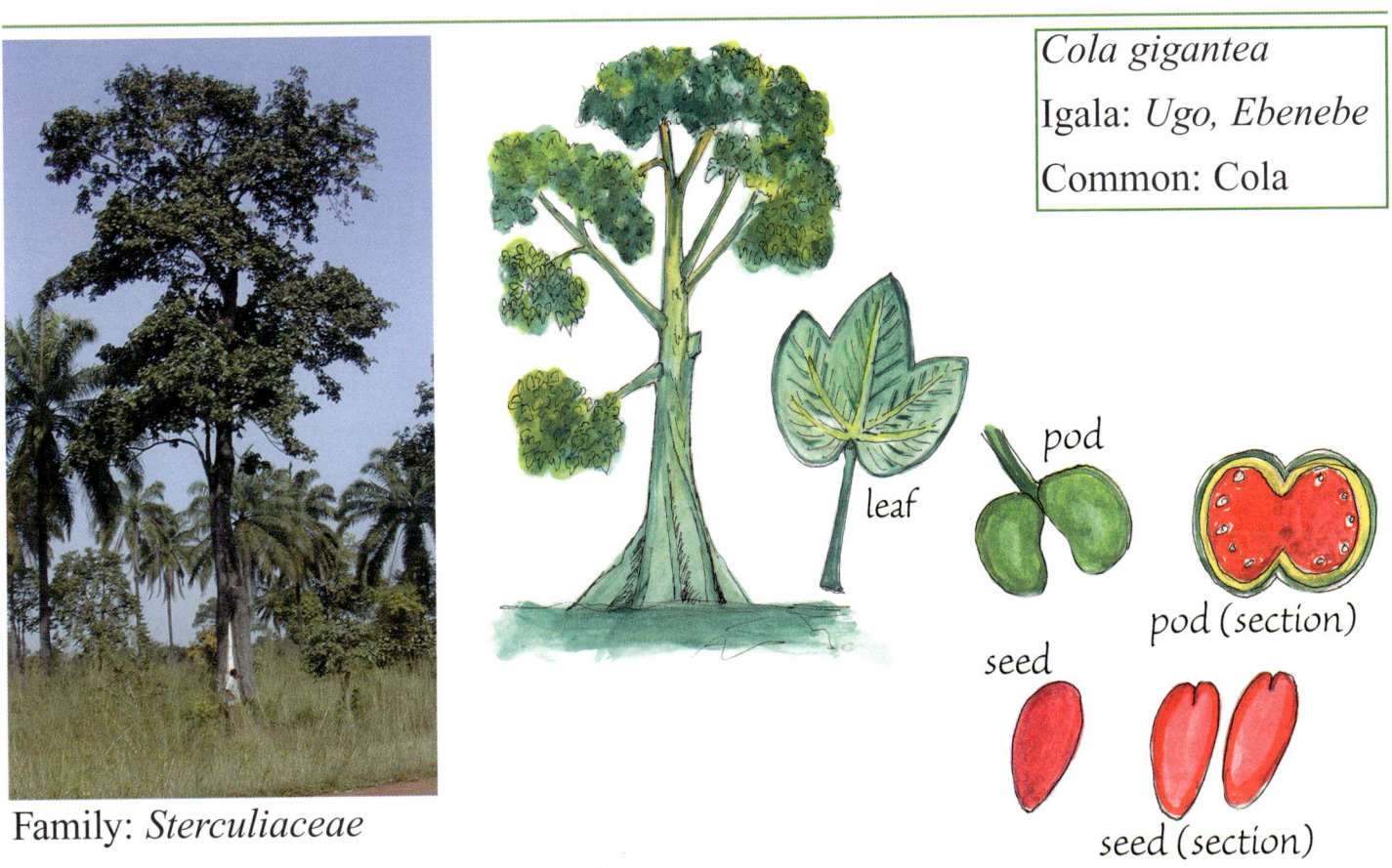

seed (section)

Family: *Sterculiaceae*

Forest tree growing up to 100 ft high. Flowers are white to pink to purple.

43

•Food

Not used as food.

•Medicinal

The bark when pounded and mixed with cold water produces a paste which cures malaria and headache.

Divide the paste, dilute with cold water and take one glass 3 times a day for 7 days. The rest of the paste can be put into a bath for the patient who enjoys immediate relief from fever.

To cure snake bites, fevers and convulsions a special formulation is recommended. Freshly peel the bark and pound to a paste with water added to make a palatable taste and texture.

The treatment can be taken orally. Dosage: 1 glass 4 times a day for 7 days and can be applied externally. If convulsions are severe take up to 5 times daily.

•Cultural

The rainmakers use it to both attract and prevent rain. The method used is their prerogative and a secret they will not reveal.

Carvers use it for idols, ornaments and other traditional images.

Tradition beliefs are that it is unsafe to shelter beneath it because if the fruit falls on your head it can result in death.

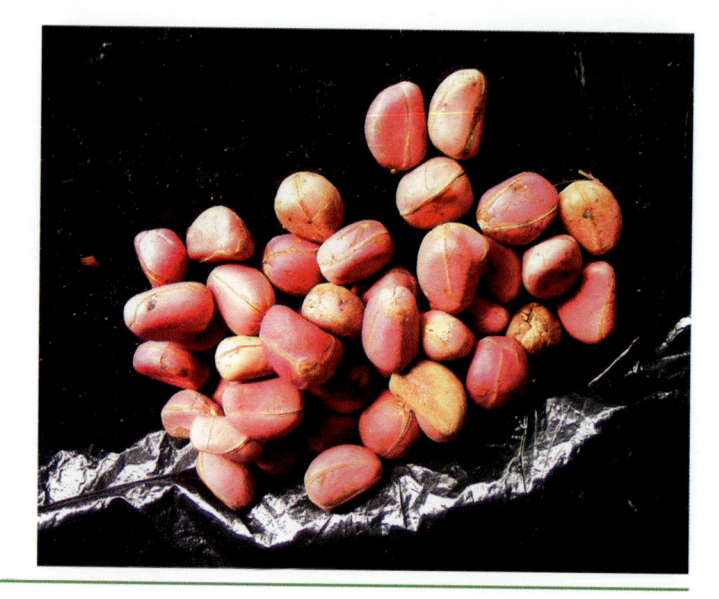

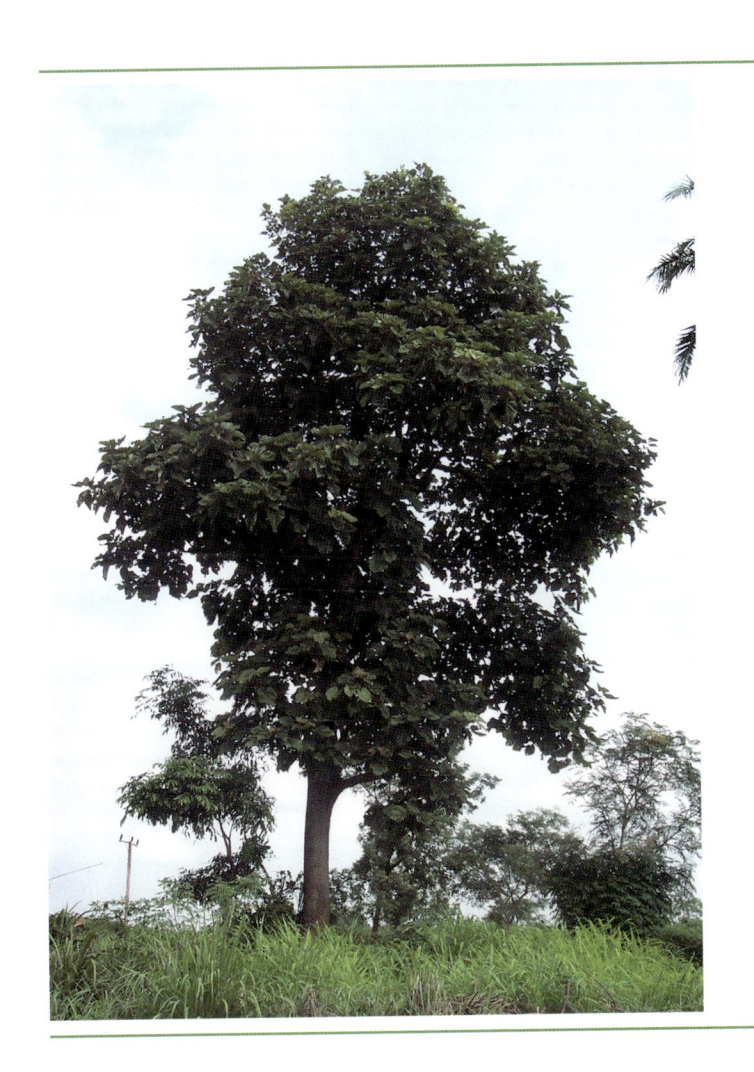

•Other uses

It once was commonly used as firewood, but now endangered, housewives and firewood dealers resort only to trees that have died.

Office and household furniture are made from it, especially tables, chairs and cupboards. Its upright trunk gives straight planks – a carpenter's dream.

Local story tellers say the tree lives for as long as 500 years.

Its fork sticks and stems are used for local buildings and its wood is generally excellent as a roofing material.

It produces abundant biomass. Despite its good shade children are scared to rest beneath it as its heavy pods cause injuries when they fall.

The bark, recognised as medicinal, provides a good source of income. The leaves, sold for the preservation of cola nuts, also fetch a tidy sum.

Cola nitida

Igala: *Obi-Akechi, Atala*

Common: Cola

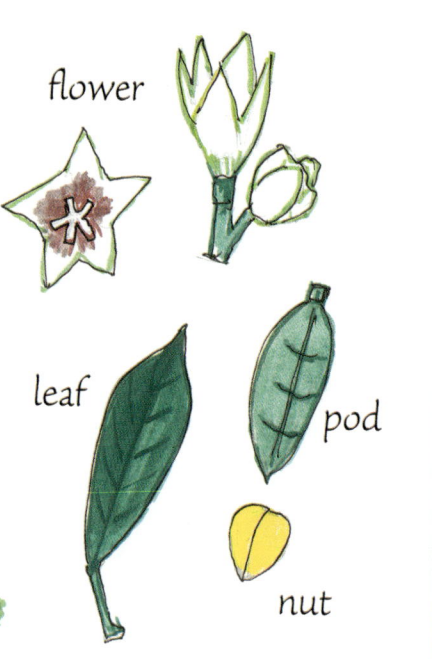

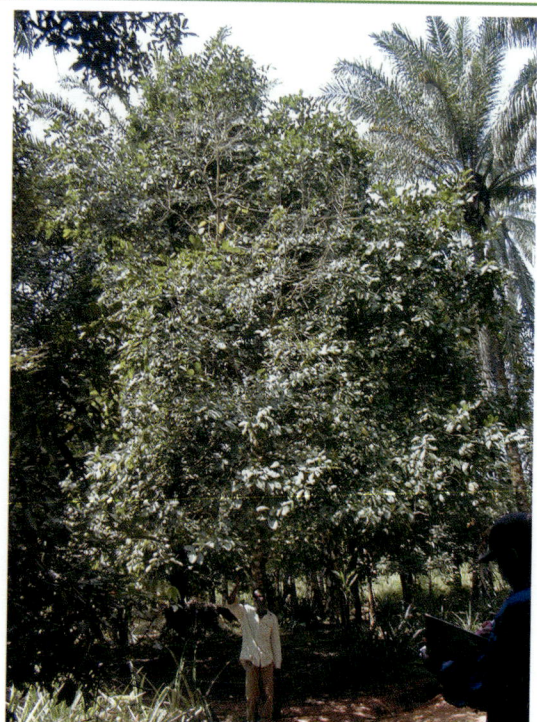

flower

leaf

pod

nut

Family: *Sterculiaceae*

Forest tree growing up to 80 ft high. Flowers are white to pink or even purple. Flowers are cream-coloured with dark reddish markings within. Often cultivated.

•Food

Obi-Atechi has no value as food, but can be chewed as a stimulant.

•Medicinal

To cure chest pain and cough, dry the cola nut, grind into powder and mix with either olive oil or honey. Take a spoon of the paste morning and evening for as long as needed.

To build up blood quickly mix the bark with tender teak and *ugbakolo* leaves. Boil in water. Cool slightly, and if possible add the blood of tortoise.

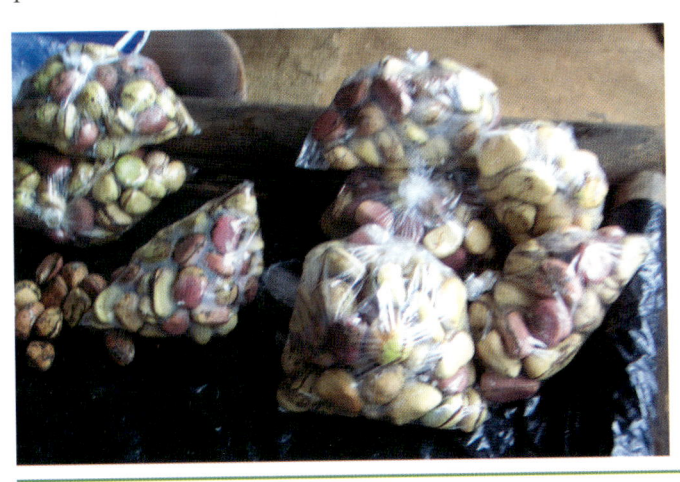

•Cultural

Culturally it enjoys most of the attributes of *Cola acuminata* except for oracle consultancy. Traditional belief is that who brings cola, brings life.

Obi-Atechi has two pairs of nuts whereas *C. accuminata* can have up to 5 pairs. For this reason it is not presented to idols. Because it is less expensive than *C. acuminata*, more people have access to it. It can be included in food celebrations and as part of prayers for progress.

•Other uses

Obi-Akechi improves soil fertility, as is evident from the picture below. Note the well established and healthy maize crop in its immediate environs.

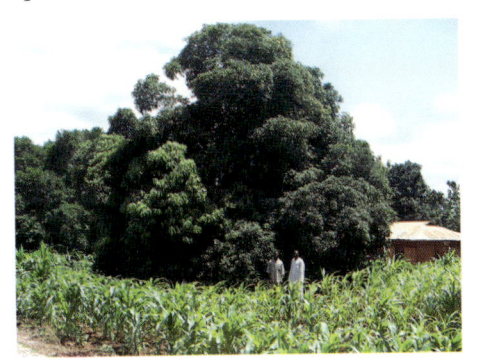

Cynometra vogelii

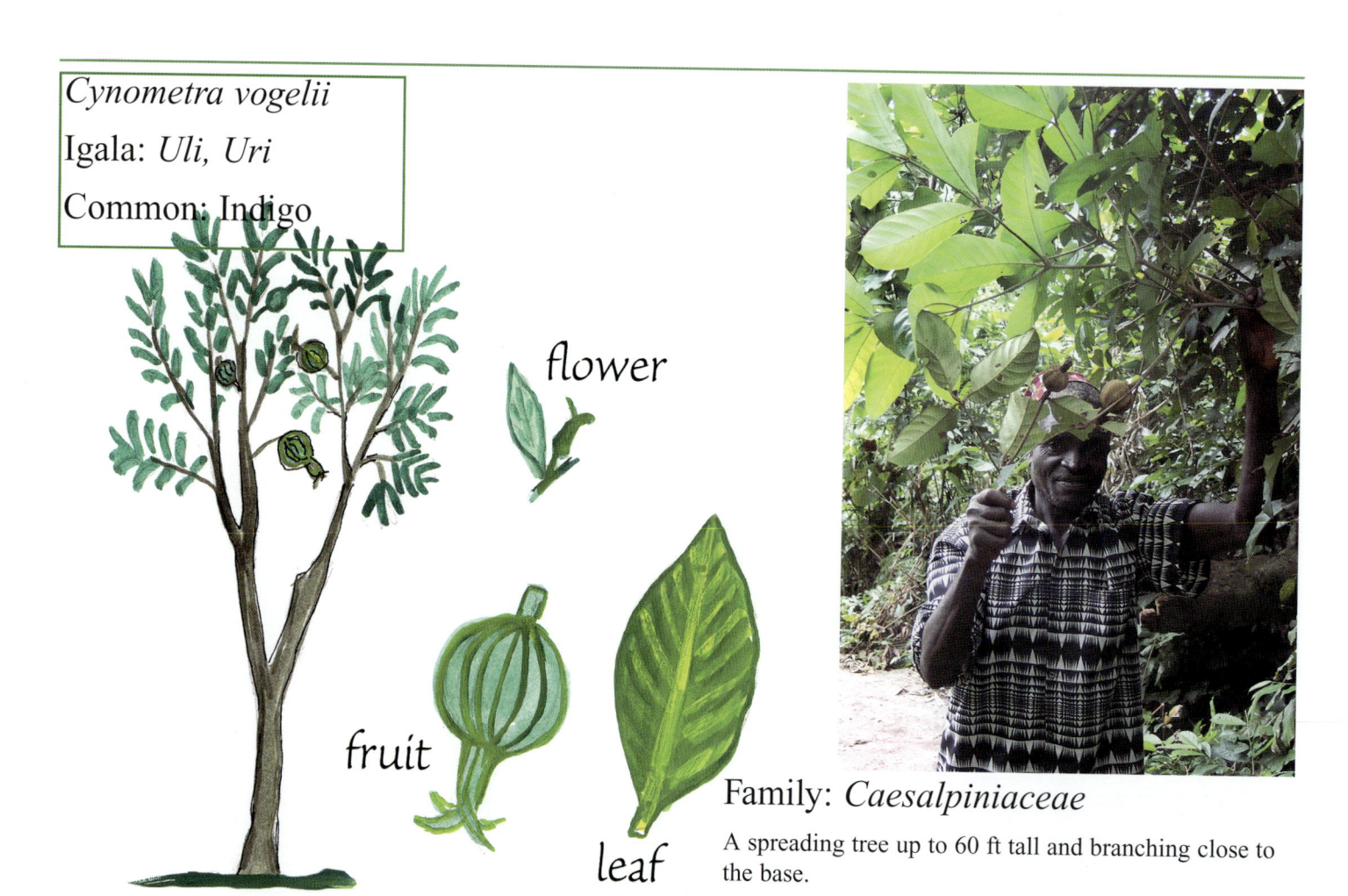

Igala: *Uli, Uri*

Common: Indigo

flower

fruit

leaf

Family: *Caesalpiniaceae*

A spreading tree up to 60 ft tall and branching close to the base.

•Food

No value as food.

•Medicinal

For impotent men: grind leaves into a paste with overripe pawpaw and take 2 glasses diluted with water 4 times a day. The leftover paste can be applied at bedtime to the body, mainly around the waist.

To treat children with measles, extract the juice from the leaves and apply to the rashes and joints.

•Cultural

As its name might suggest its primary use is as a dye. The fresh leaves and fruit when ground together turn into black ink used for dying clothes and making designs on plain cloth.

Women use it for beautification marks on their face, arms and legs, especially for dancing festivals. Elders and idol worshippers decorate their idols with it.

In olden days, when feuds were common, warriors disguised themselves by applying it to their faces and bodies.

During local festivals (*Ogani Angwa*), people still apply it to disguise themselves.

Nowadays as the tree is endangered, a blue dye and local chalk (*afu*) serve as an alternative.

Muslims use it instead of chalk for writing on boards when teaching the Koran.

•Other uses

Indigo is regarded as a cash crop and its seed sold in most markets.

Farm tools and axe holders, important implements in the farming communities in the region, are sometimes made from it.

Alternatives will be found as the seeds become more valuable.

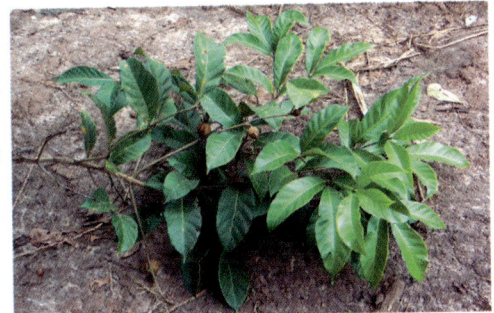

Daniellia oliveri

Igala: *Agba, Akpachi*

Common: African Copaiba Balsam Tree, West African Gum Copal

leaf

flower

branch

seed

seed

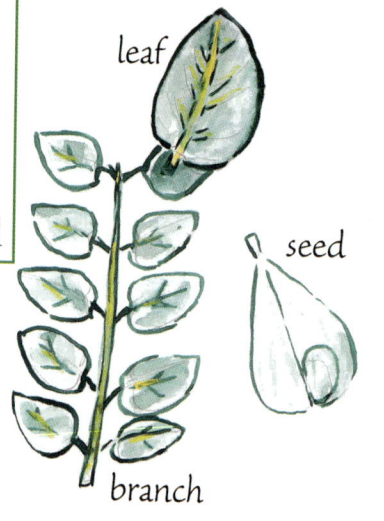

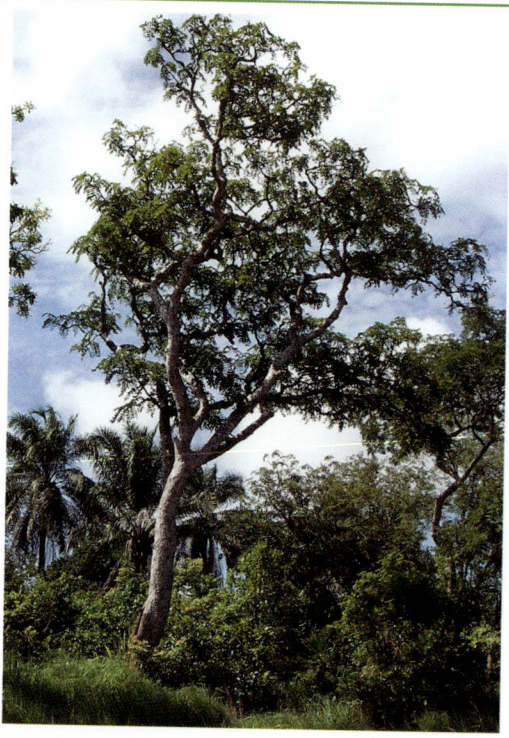

Family: *Caesalpiniaceae*

A savannah tree growing up to 100 ft tall with white scented flowers and smooth, pale and flat seeds.

- **Food**

The mushroom which grows on it is enjoyed as a vegetable.

- **Medicinal**

To cure malaria, the bark is ground to a paste using water. The paste when diluted with either hot or cold water is given to the patient in 1 glass twice daily for 7 days.

To cure backache, paste made from the bark is applied externally to the part which aches. Water can be added to the paste and 1 glass taken 3 times daily for 7 days. This liquid formulation treats typhoid, stomach pain and dysentery in similar doses.

To cure headache, stomach ache and typhoid fever, pound the bark to a paste, mould into small round portions. Once dried, grind and dilute with cold water. Dosage: 1 glass, twice daily for 7 days.

- **Cultural**

The tree mostly found close to the village provides a traditional worshipping site.

- **Other uses**

Unfortunately, the *agba* is now an endangered species but when ever possible can still be used for roofing, domestic and office furniture, farm tools and axe handles. Local games are still made from it.

The soil also benefits from its presence.

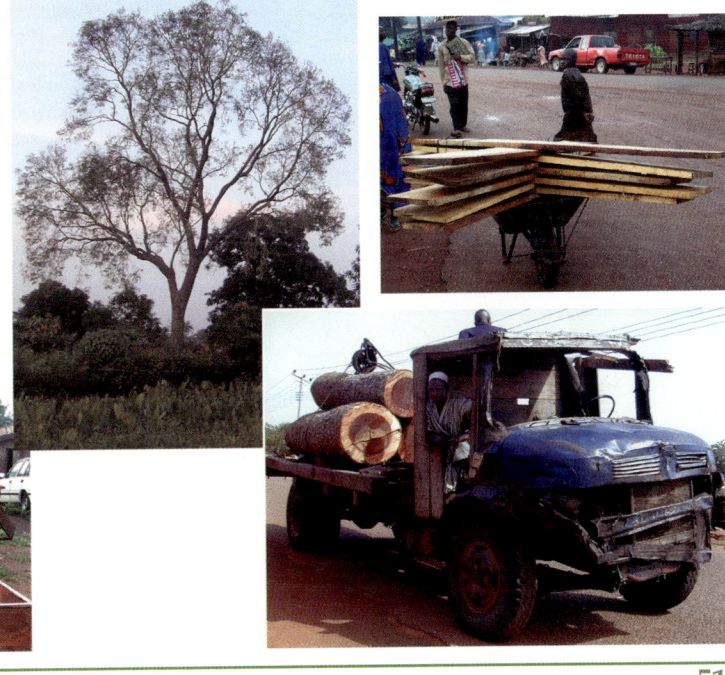

Dialium guineense

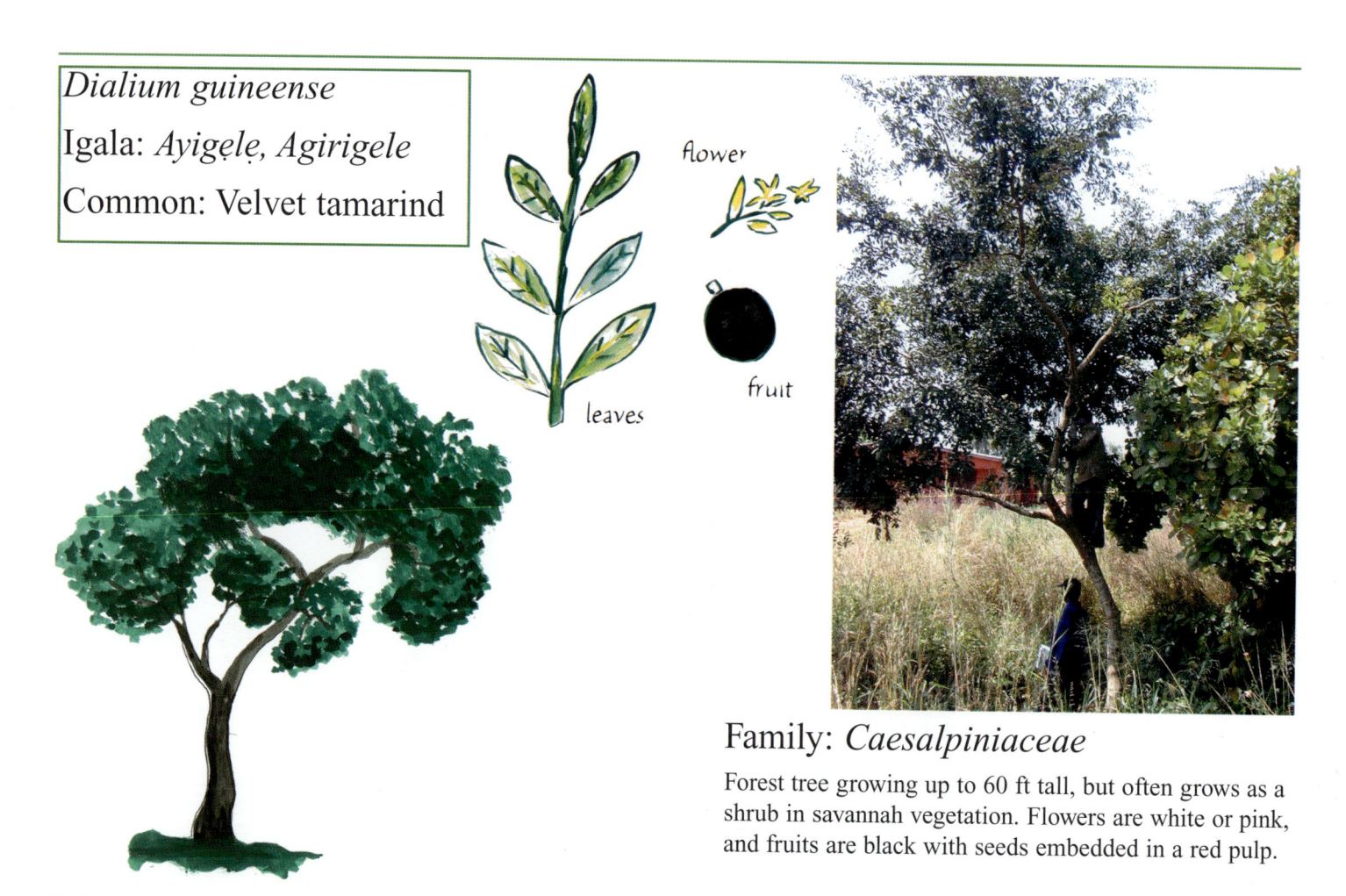

Igala: *Ayigẹlẹ, Agirigele*

Common: Velvet tamarind

leaves

flower

fruit

Family: *Caesalpiniaceae*

Forest tree growing up to 60 ft tall, but often grows as a shrub in savannah vegetation. Flowers are white or pink, and fruits are black with seeds embedded in a red pulp.

•Food

Its tender leaves serve as an ingredient for vegetable soup. Fruits can be eaten raw.

•Medicinal

To treat malaria fever and all bodily pains, its leaves are added to lemon and *ogẹlẹ* leaves and boiled; some of the potion can be taken orally and some reserved for bathing.

To cure nausea during pregnancy, add black pepper to tamarind leaf and boil in water; take while still warm. Dosage: 1 glass 3 times daily for 7 days.

The ground tamarind leaf can be taken raw for coughs and vomiting.

Those suffering from stroke can be cured if the bark is ground to a paste, then divided and part applied externally. The rest when diluted with cold or warm water can be taken in the most common measure of: 1 glass, 3 times daily for 7 days.

To cure vomiting in children boil the leaves and give a spoonful of the potion to the child 4 to 5 times daily until better. The same medicine can be given to children with measles, but the dosage is 1 glass 3 times daily until better (may take up to 2 weeks).

Also good for chest pain and cough, but in the latter case *akamu* (corn porridge) is added.

•Cultural

No cultural use in the region.

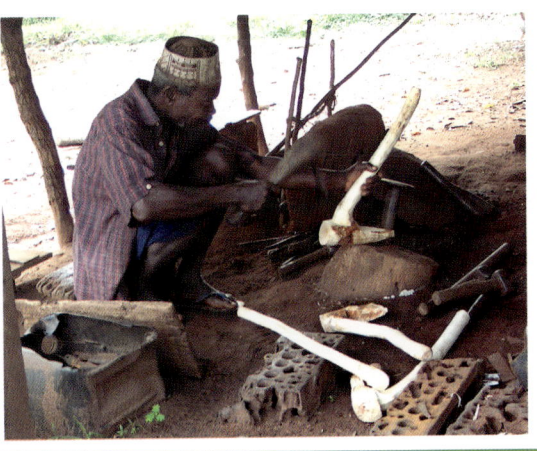

•Other uses

Commonly used to make handles for farm tools.

It is well known to improve soil fertility

Its pretty flower adds colour to the many shades of green in the panorama.

Ekebergia senegalensis

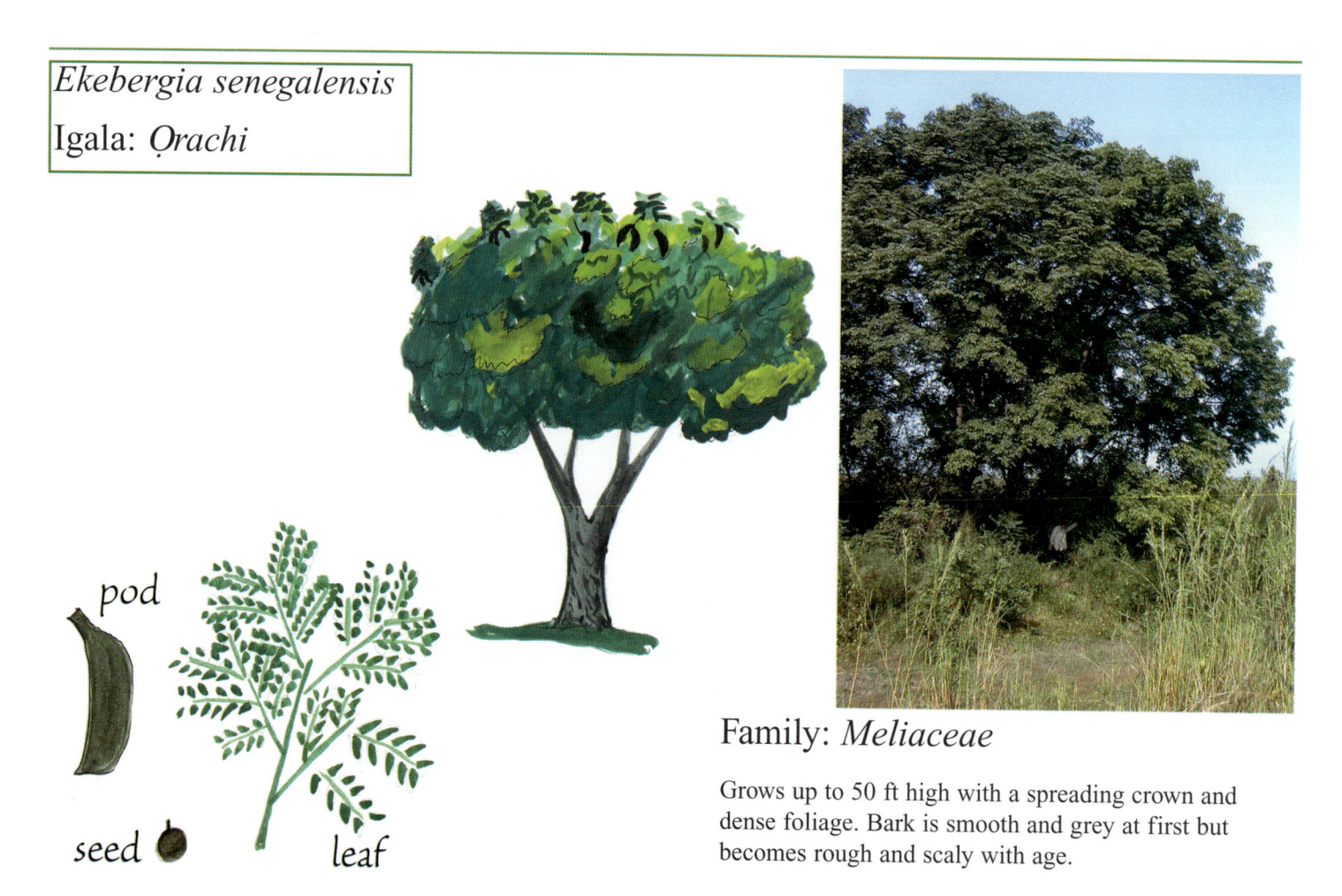

Igala: *Ọrachi*

pod

seed

leaf

Family: *Meliaceae*

Grows up to 50 ft high with a spreading crown and dense foliage. Bark is smooth and grey at first but becomes rough and scaly with age.

- **Food**

The Ọrachi tree has nothing edible.

- **Medicinal**

The medicinal form of *Ọrachi* can cure jaundice. Boil its leaves with those of guava and sugar cane. Cool slightly. Drink while still warm. Dosage: 1 glass 3 times daily for 7 days.

When the leaves and bark are boiled together the formulation is used in the treatment of epilepsy. Dosage: 1 glass of cooled liquid 3 times daily for 7 days. After this the medicine has to be made afresh.

For the treatment of wounds believed to be the work of witches and wizards, the *Ọrachi* leaves and bark are ground together into a paste. The paste is then applied to affected parts after they have been cleaned and washed with the medicine from the boiled leaf and bark. This is done 3 times daily for 7 days. 3 - 4 rounds of treatment may be needed if the wounds are serious.

All types of wound can be treated with *Ọrachi*. The bark boiled in water is generally used for washing the wound.

- **Cultural**

Since the shade of an *Ọrachi* tree constitutes a worshipping site with ancestors residing beneath, it is therefore considered dangerous. Their presence therefore would make it uncomfortable for witches, wizards and devils to come there.

In olden days people accused of being witches were tried by the *Ọrachi* bark. The leaves and bark were ground with water into a paste and if the accused vomited the paste and survived then his/her name was cleared. Failing this the person died and went to the grave stigmatized.

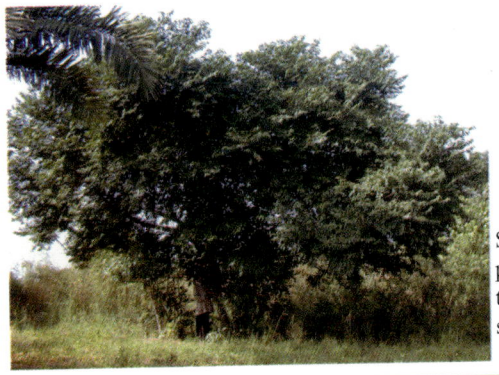

Soil benefits from its presence as can be seen from the luscious growth surrounding it in this picture

When you make a fire with Ọrachi it drives away bad spirits from the compound.

Watch out! There are two Ọrachi – one poisonous, the other benign and used for medicine. The poisonous Ọrachi akpula is not selective, and should anyone ever consume the paste from its leaves and bark, death is certain. Few take the chance as the two trees are practically identical.

Pictured are handles for agricultural implements - good examples of local industries central to the farming community that owe their existence to Ọrachi.

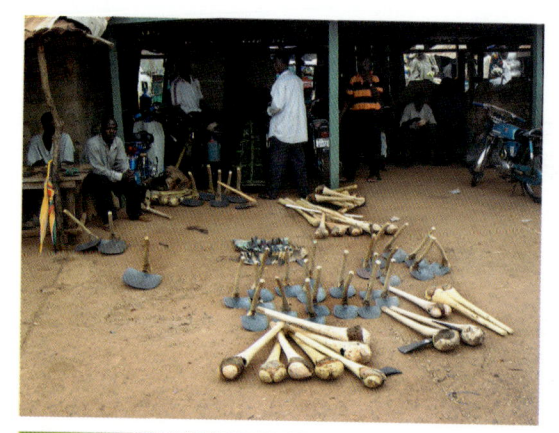

•Other uses

As firewood it burns for long, but now endangered and therefore seen as something of a luxury. Its charcoal is as good as its firewood.

Sturdy in stature it produces even stronger wood than Iroko. It has to be well seasoned for three to four years before use, after which it resembles iron. Not surprisingly it is the main tree used for canoe and boat making, with canoes said to last for 150 to 200 years.

Excellent for the construction of roofs, local housing and granaries, and as handles for farm tools.

A best bet as a cash crop. It is the most expensive of all timber in the region, the reason being that chain saw operators charge highly for cutting it, especially the well seasoned iron-like type.

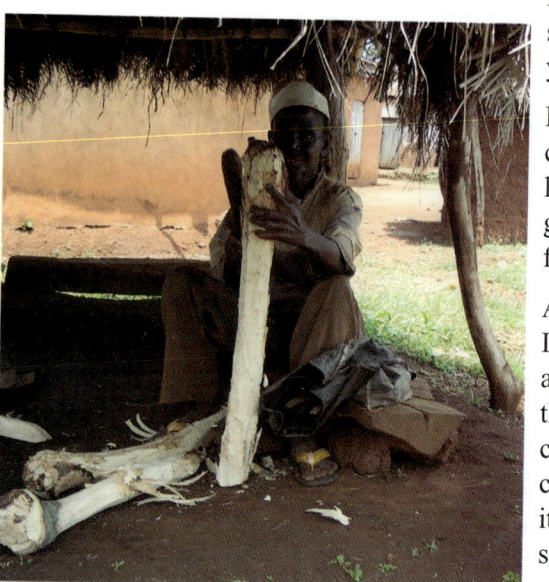

Elaeis guineensis

Igala: *Ẹkpẹ*

Common: Oil palm

fruit

tree

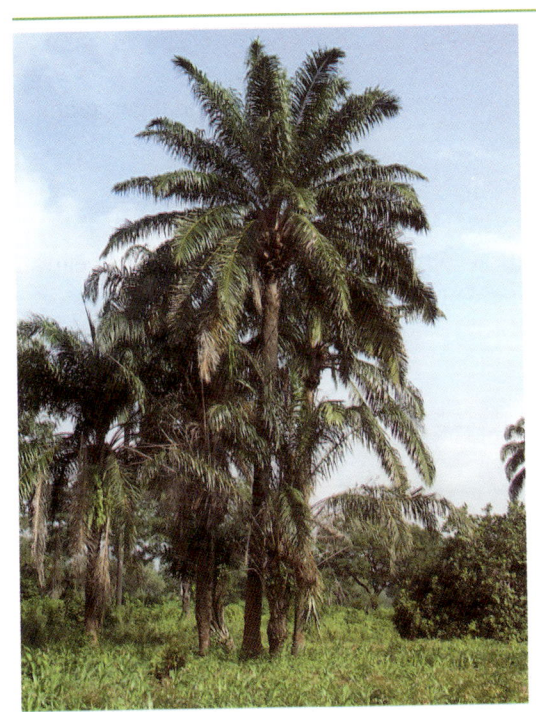

leaf frond

bunch

Family: *Palmae*

Grows up to 20m tall; straight trunk with arching dark-green leaves, 4 - 5m long. Both male and female flowers on the same tree; fruits grow in clusters known as bunches, weighing 3 - 15kg. One of the most important trees in the area.

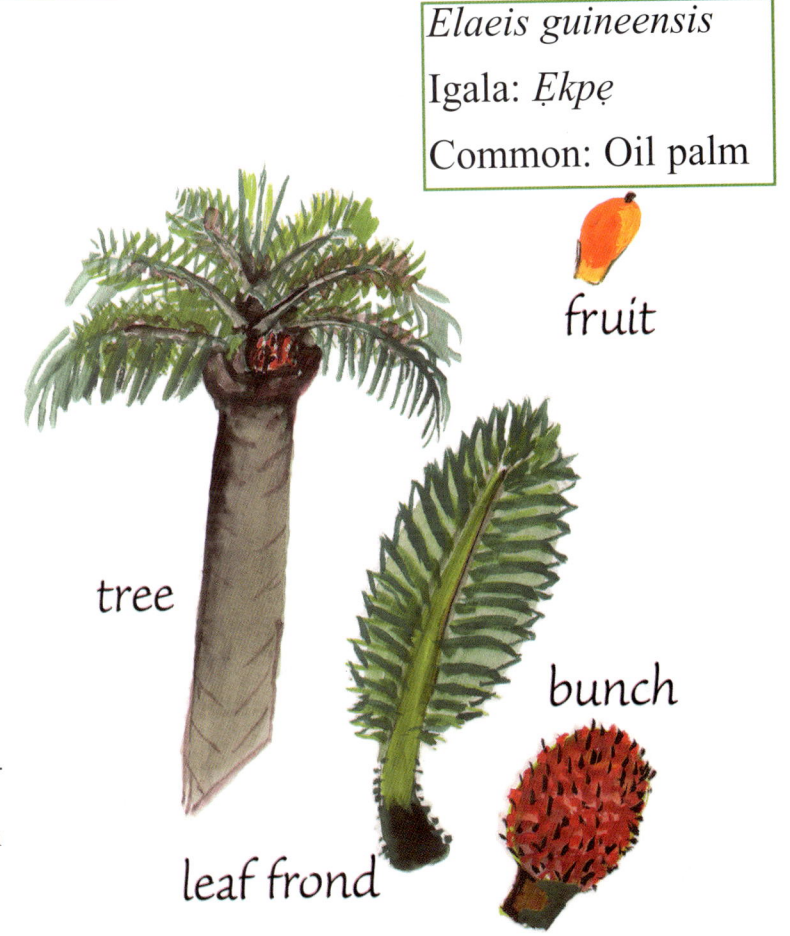

This valuable natural resource has many purposes requiring different skills and indigenous knowledge passed from one generation to the next. All parts of the tree are extremely useful but the three main products obtained from it are palm wine, palm oil and palm kernel oil (pko).

Palm wine is the sap of the male flower (inflorescence) only. This (unfermented) 'wine' is obtained through a process known as tapping.

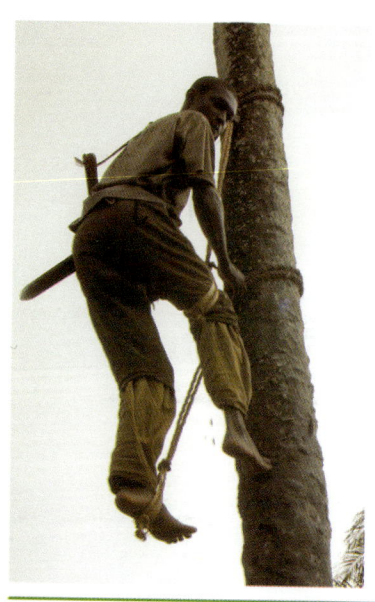

A tapper climbs the tree, inserts tubing, connected to a container, into a slit at the base of the the male flower. The container gradually fills with the 'wine'. Tapping just 2 litres a day ensures the tree will continue to produce both palm fruit and wine. Less sustainable methods, would result in the early death of the tree.

The special implements for tapping wine and cutting bunches are made by local blacksmiths.

Both tappers and harvesters use the same type of rope and methods of tree climbing. The rope is also made from the tree. These skills are passed from one generation to the next and belong to a small percentage of the population. Both activities are expensive because of the dangers involved. 'No one ever fell from a palm tree and lived normally afterwards', they say.

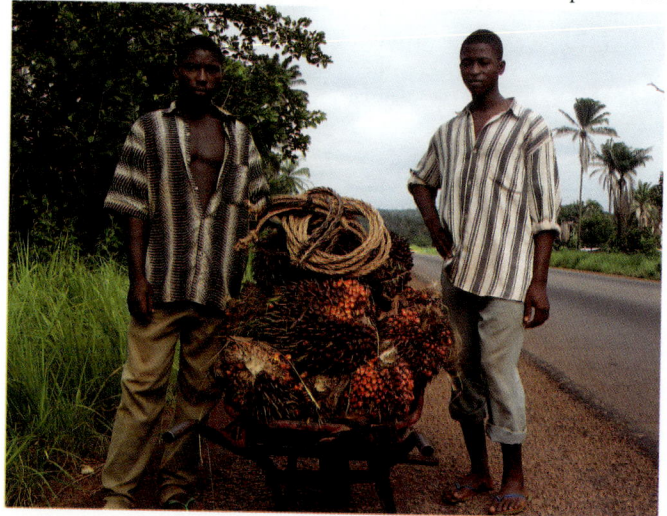

Ropes and bunches of mature palm fruit

Palm wine and other drinks made from it are the main alcoholic beverages in this area. It is not potent immediately after tapping but the level of alcohol increases as it ferments. Local distilleries turn palm wine into local gin (80-100% alcohol content) with a minimum of equipment and expense.

To produce local gin the 'wine' is left to ferment in a drum for 4-5 days before being transferred to another drum which is then placed over a fire. As the temperature gradually rises to 100 °c the liquid transforms into vapour. This vapour then passes through a pipe, which runs through a container filled with cold water, to its final destination called the collector. The middle drum of cold water acts as a coolant which turns the vapour back to a liquid.

This process of Fractional Distillation is not known as such by the women who are adept at this work. Though a major source of income for women who enjoy complete monopoly of the trade, they never consume it. This local gin is cheaper than beer or palm wine and only a little is needed to become intoxicated.

Because of its capacity to intoxicate it has many nicknames such as *Kayi-Kayi* (push me, push you) and *Ikpa maji* (if it kills you they will bury you).

Also known as Sapẹlẹ water, it is now more popularly known as *ogogoro*, its original name when first introduced from Sapẹlẹ, Delta State, where the practice originated. Another is *agwugwuyee* or *ote-ajalu*, meaning a silent drink that intoxicates more than others that make noise. Tasting like strong western gin, drinks referred to locally as 'hot', it is often said that Kayi-Kayi is 'hot very well'. Another is *adononojo dọmanẹ*, meaning if you drink enough you behave like the locals. Yet another name is *ọgbakala* – it changes an elder to a child – enough said!

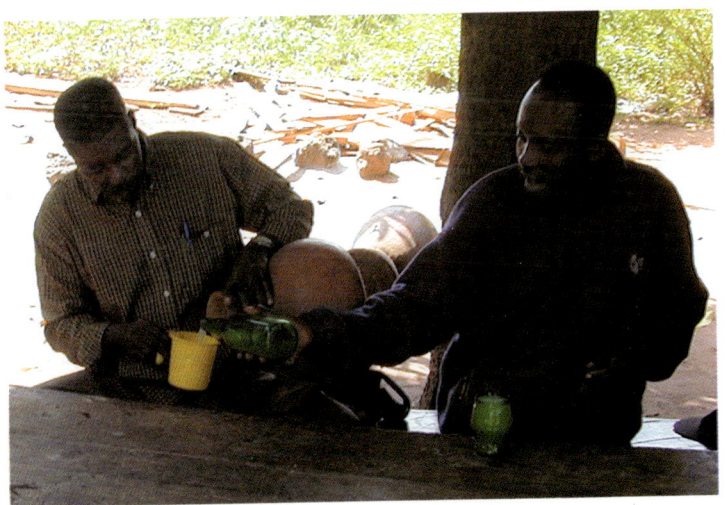

Men relaxing with a glass of palm wine or gin

To date elders have not changed their practice of honouring their ancestors. Even with the advent of western drink they still use palm wine and *kayi kayi*.

Palm wine and palm oil are an important part of the tithes paid to traditional leaders.

Palm oil production is a more 'sober' business than local gin production and, like the production of local gin, it too is completely in the hands of women.

Men play a key role in producing the tree, but women are in charge of producing the oil. However, palm bunches are one of the few farm products sold by men, with women often buying bunches from the men for their own palm oil business. However, there are various traditions surrounding the supply of bunches and the production of palm oil for household use. Generally husbands are responsible for supplying bunches to their wives who produce the palm oil free of charge on behalf of the household. All residues from this process are the property of the wives.

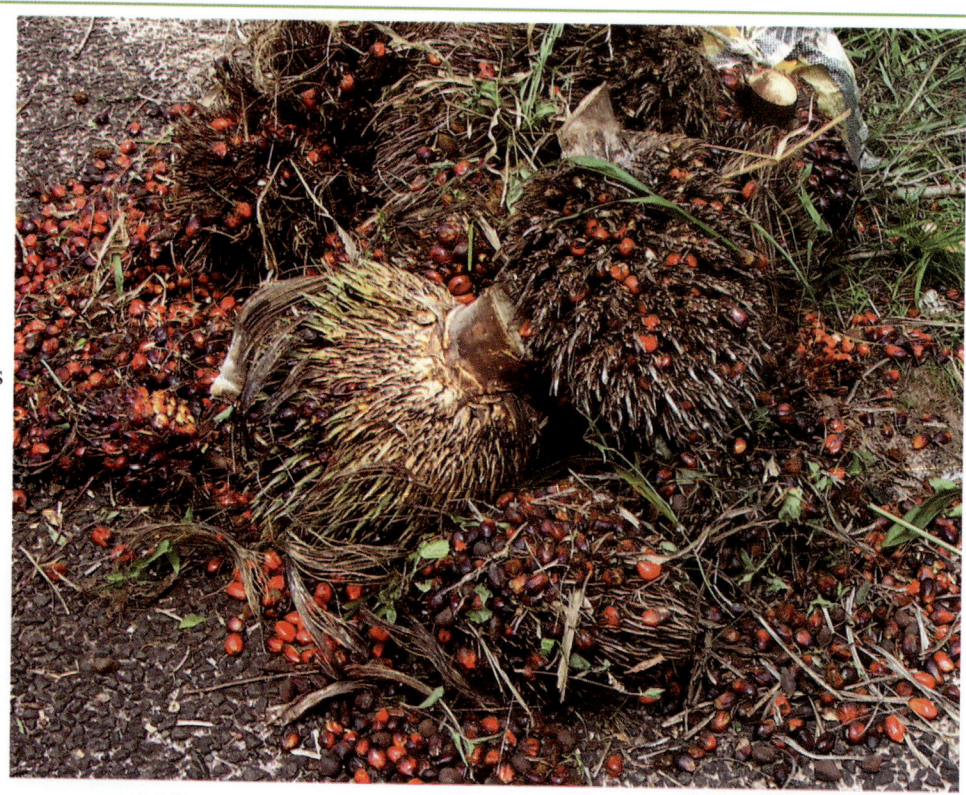

Freshly harvested bunches of palm fruit

Palm oil production is laborious, involving days of hard work and energy.

The freshly harvested bunches are collected in wheelbarrows and brought to the place of processing. The palm bunches are then cooked in black drums as can be seen in the picture below. It also shows nuts already cooked and separated from the bunch.

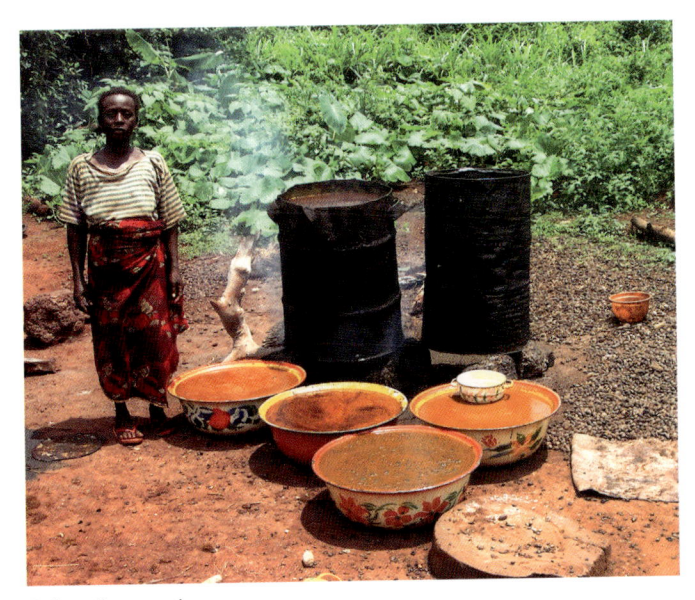

Palm oil extraction

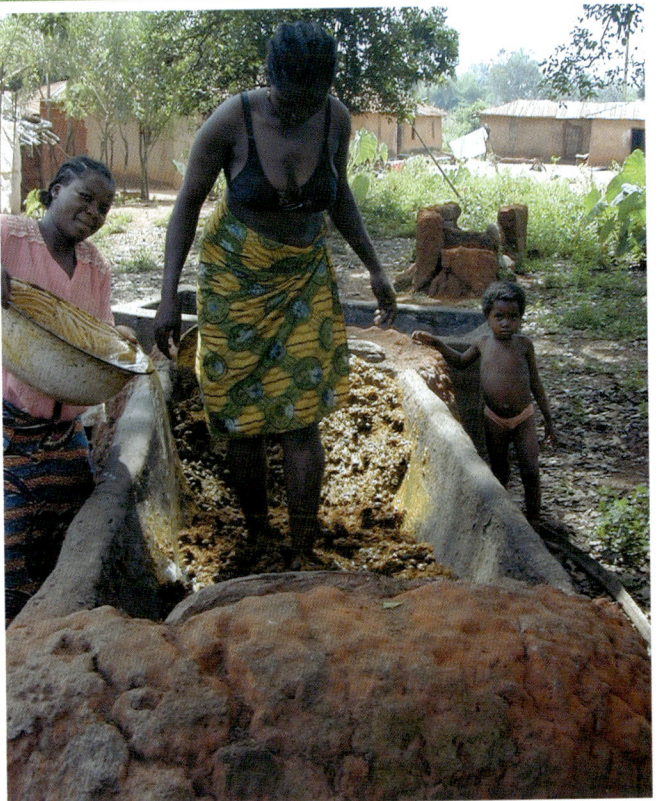

Above the trough (*agwu*) where the women pound the cooked nuts to which water has been added. This produces palm oil and also separates the kernel from the flesh of the fruit. This kernel is then used for pko.

•Cultural

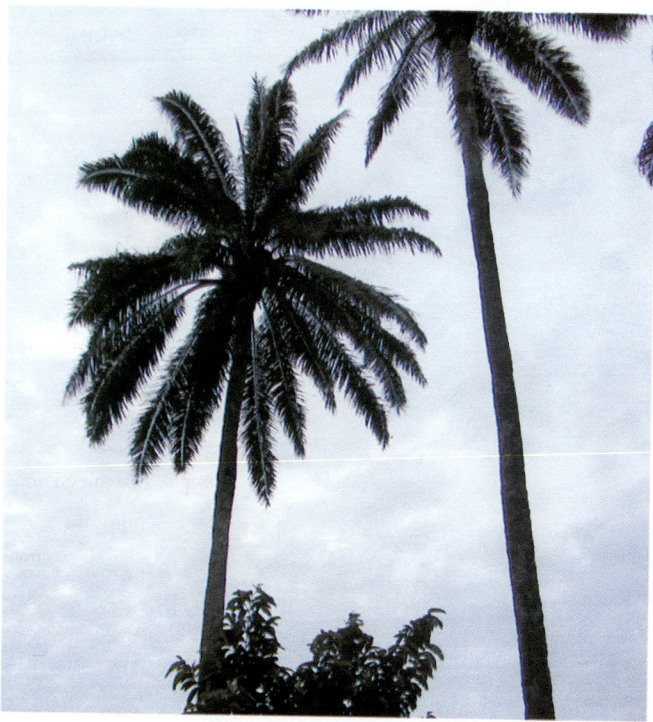

This majestic yet unassuming tree is the symbol of Igalaland - an institution in its own right, surrounded and protected by a legal system.

Palm oil is obtained by extracting the oil from the freshly harvested ripe bunches of palm fruits, a lengthy process taking several days.

Palm kernel oil (pko) is the oil made from the kernel left after the oil has been extracted from the flesh. This is also a lengthy process whereby the nut (kernel), which is contained in the palm fruit, is turned into oil.

Two types of pko are manufactured from palm kernel. For the first type the oil is extracted by burning the kernel, for the second the oil is extracted by pounding the nut. The second method is preferred because the oil produced this way is odourless and clearer. Pko, as well as being in high demand locally, is also exported.

Palm fruit (cross-section)

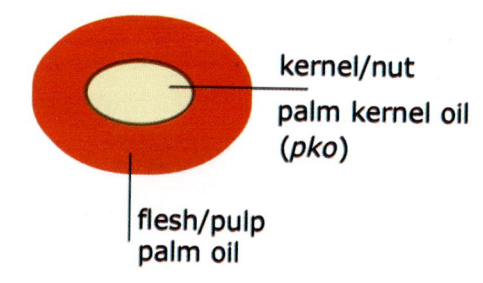

- kernel/nut
- palm kernel oil (*pko*)
- flesh/pulp palm oil

In ancestral worship palm oil is offered to idols, but palm kernel oil is never allowed near them as they fear it might kill them. However, palm wine is presented to the ancestors through their idols.

Palm wine accompanies cola nut in all stages of a marriage ceremony and is meant to give a sense of belonging.

• Food

The palm kernel nut is edible in its raw state. Palm fruit is eaten raw in combination with gari (cassava), or roasted and eaten on its own.

Palm oil is used in almost all Igala soups (stew – obo).

• Other uses

A by-product of the palm oil industry is an oily fibrous substance which when dried is used to kindle fires, replacing Kerosene.

Oil made from palm kernel, although now costly, is still cheaper than other vegetable oils produced locally or imported.

Palm kernel is expensive because it is used in the local manufacture of cosmetics, soaps and candles. Kernels are now coveted as an export crop.

Every part of the oil palm tree is good for use as firewood, especially when dead. Even a dead palm is valuable.

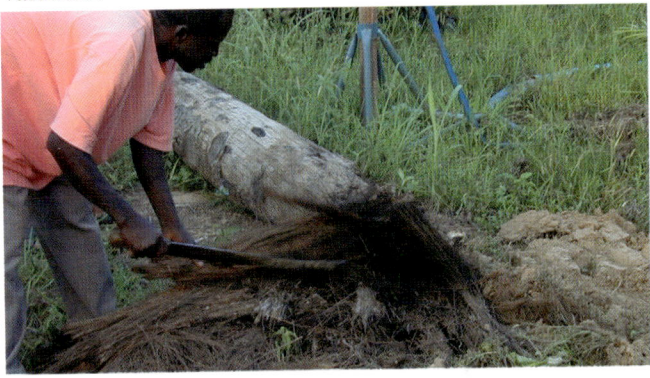

A dead tree being cut into smaller pieces and applied as mulch and compost

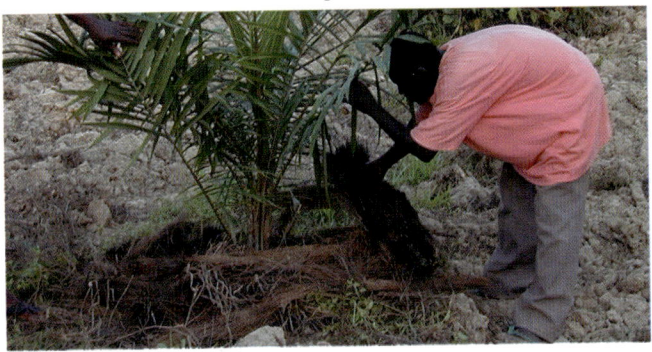

Some residues are richer than others. The residue from the 'cooked' bunches and inflorescents, for example, is rich in potassium. When applied to fruit trees, particularly oranges, the result is excellent fruit formation and sweeter fruits, giving higher market value.

Palm fronds make good roofs, birdcages and fish traps.

Matches, baskets, fans, fences, ceilings, temporary canopies, local bathrooms, brooms, local beds and doors are also made from palm fronds.

Its leaflets are also used for making frames for local farm buildings and dwellings for animals. Drums made from them are not too popular because of their weight.

The oil palm has long been acknowledged as one of the best enhancers of soil fertility. Providing the best shade in the forest, it also destroys many weeds. Wild birds nest in it.

The tree is magnificent and depicts the beauty, romantic and exotic in the African panorama.

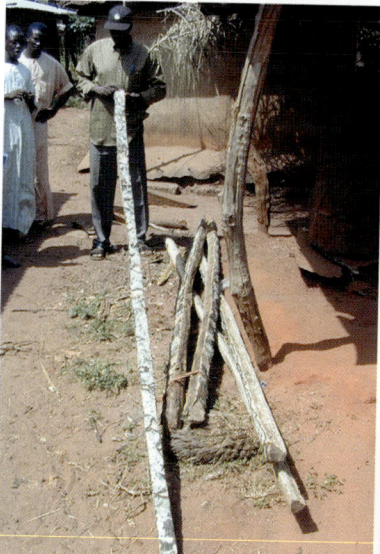

Ribs from palm fronds used for buildings

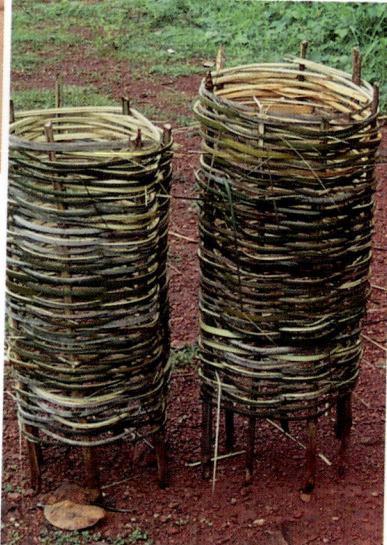

Seedling guards provide protection from goats

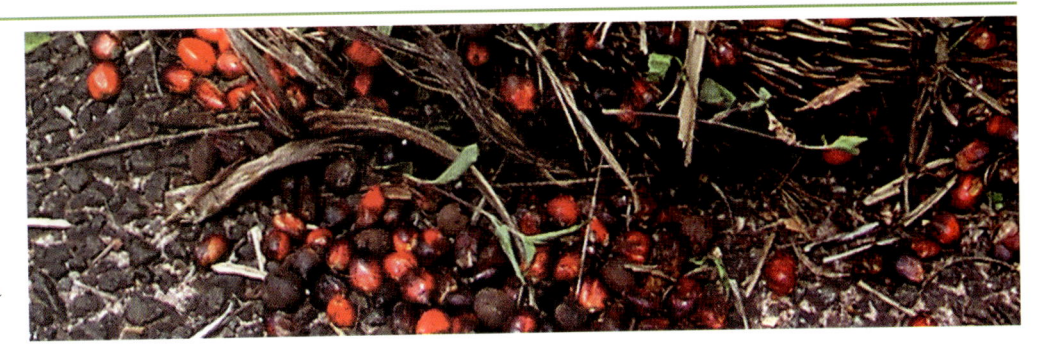

•Medicinal

To cure typhoid take a quarter of a glass of pko daily for 7 days.

Pko is added to many prescriptions to counteract poison. It is also included in potions to cure convulsions, headache and meningitis.

To combat general skin disease including eczema, Pko, *akalipa* (a flower used in treating skin disease), gunpowder and *ogwujęba* are mixed together and applied externally.

Children and adults with stomach ache, typhoid and constipation also take pko. Dosage: 2 spoonfuls 3 times daily for 7 days.

For poison mistakenly swallowed, palm oil is taken as an antidote. Traditionally 1-2 Peak milk tins-full are taken every 2 hours. This induces vomiting which gets rid of the poison.

Another treatment for poisoning is to boil the bark and use some of the water for bathing. Immediately after bathing, the remainder is given at the common dosage rate of 1 glass 3 times daily for 7 days.

To cure dysentery and diarrhoea, the leaves of palm, *ogichi* and *ikękęnę* are boiled and drunk while warm. Dosage: 1 glass 3 times daily for 7 days. To cure diarrhoea more effectively, *akamu* (maize porridge or custard) is added to the formulation at the same dosage.

Palm wine is the major ingredient in the treatment of poison, snake bite and stroke. It also improves lactation for breast-feeding mothers.

Erythrina senegalensis

Igala: *Achęchę*

Common: Coral Flower

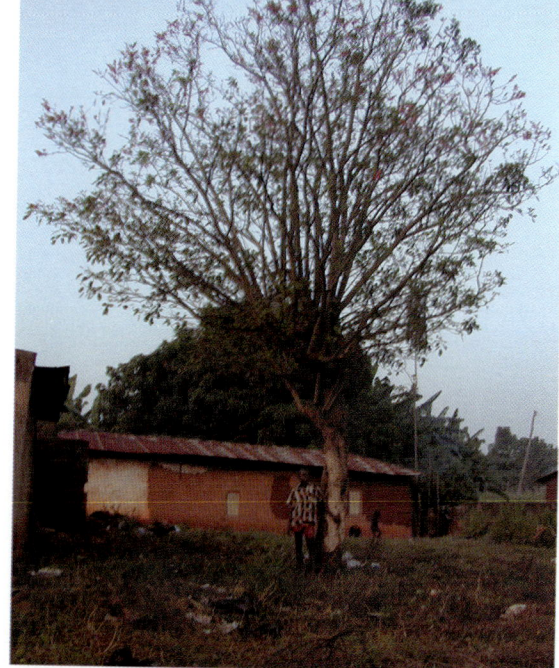

leaf

Family: *Papilionaceae*.

Usually grows as a small tree with a maximum height of 50 ft. Has stout prickles. Flowers are scarlet and usually form when tree is leafless. Commonly planted as a hedge.

•Food

It has no fruit or edible part.

•Medicinal

Patients with cough and asthma are helped by the bark. To make the potion cut the bark into pieces, place in a pot without water over a fire. This produces charcoal. Next grind into powder and add palm oil. A few spoonfuls of this syrup is given to the patients 3 times daily for 7 days.

For skin rashes apply the syrup on the affected area for as long as required.

•Cultural

Traditional believers use it as a worshipping site and place their idols beneath it.

It also serves as a live fence to demarcate plots and graves.

•Other uses

Achẹchẹ was once good for firewood but can no longer be used because it has joined the list of endangered trees.

Yam barns and granaries are still constructed from its wood. The *atakpa*, the parlour where 'strangers' (visitors) are welcomed, was also made from it. Such a building has to be sturdy as there are always activities in compounds.

Handles for axes, cutlasses and hoes were produced from it. It improves soil fertility.

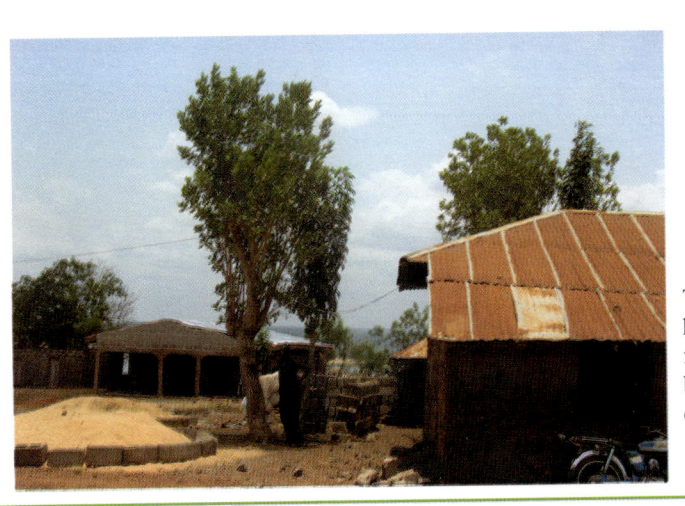

The picture highlights its use as a fence where the new building site is clearly marked.

Ficus capensis

Igala: Ọgbaikolo, Ugbakolo, Ọgbaikolo

Common: Fig tree

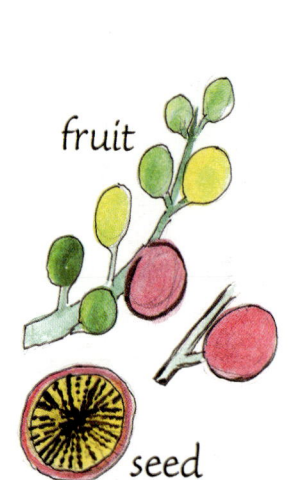

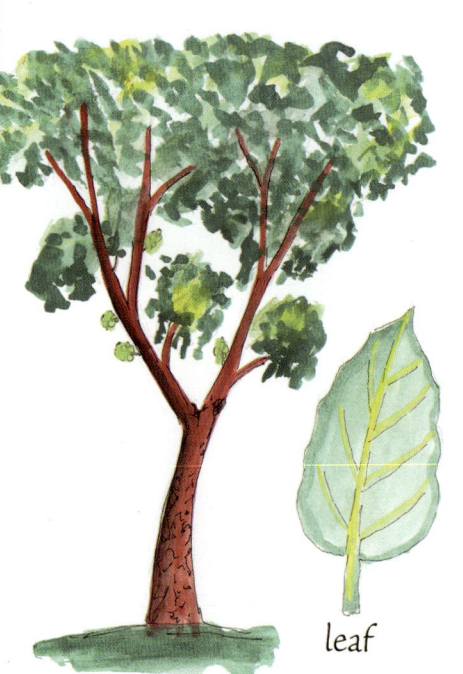

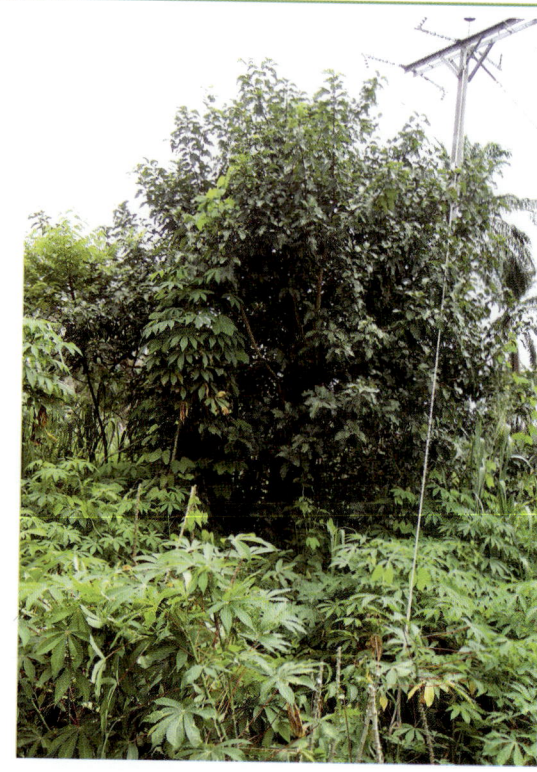

fruit

seed

leaf

Family: *Moraceae*

Usually a small tree with the figs borne as abundant clusters on the trunk. Variable in form, and common in more open country

•Food

Its leaves are good for vegetable soup and its edible fruit eaten by children.

•Medicinal

Blood tonic is made from *ugbakolo* and tender teak leaves. These are soaked in water and 1 glass taken 3 times daily for 7 days.

Typhoid, malaria fever and jaundice are cured by a similar treatment and dosage. For dysentery add guava leaf.

•Cultural

Children catch birds beneath it. Birds like its sweet fruit and tiny seeds.

Ugbakolo: Olikimabun kiya ro ulaka ulaka
A type of tree without flowers that brings forth fruit.

•Other uses

Unfortunately this tree is now endangered but if it ever becomes available it is welcome firewood.

No one questions its capacity to improve soil fertility. The picture on the previous page shows healthy plants of cassava that have benefited from its biomass.

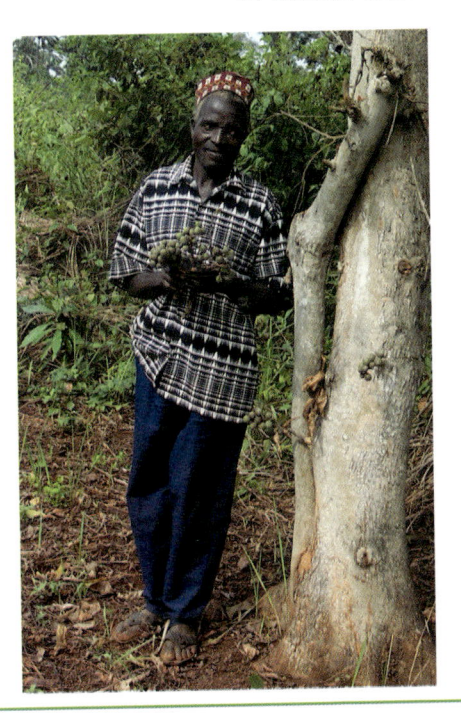

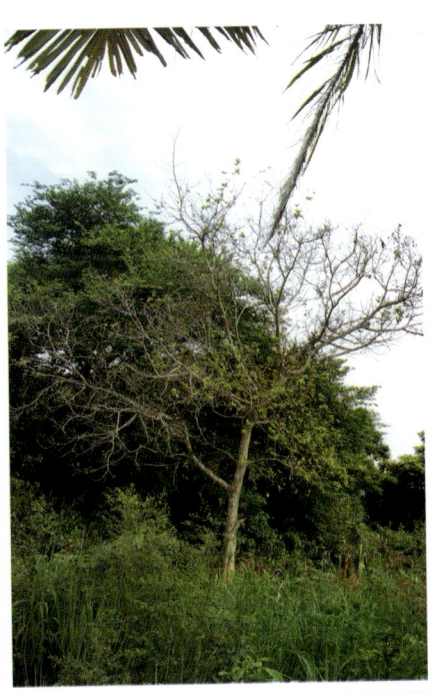

Ficus thonningii

Igala: Ọda, Ọgbu

Common: Chinese banyan, Malayan banyan, Indian laurel

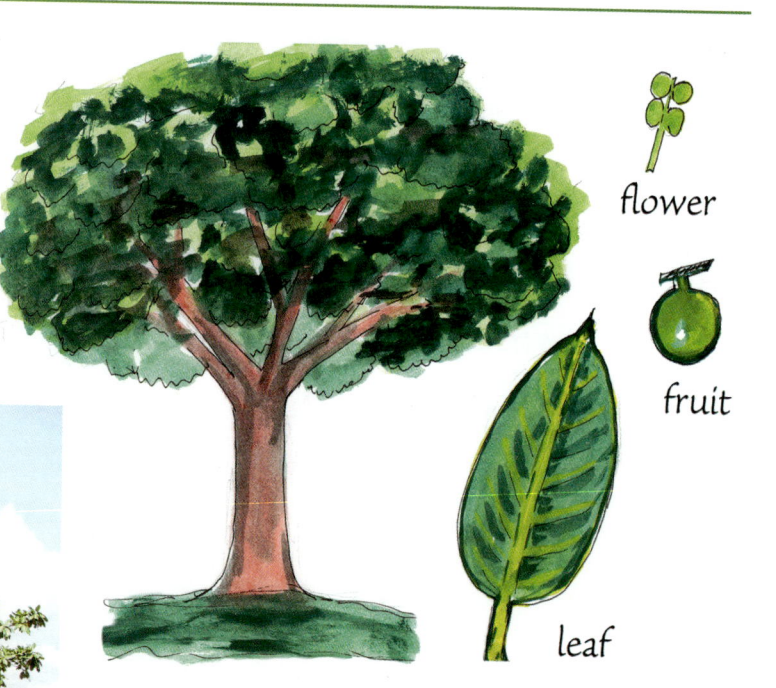

flower

fruit

leaf

Family: *Moraceae*

Tree up to 60 ft tall with dark green foliage and numerous aerial roots. Often planted near compounds for shade.

- **Food**

Leaves are used to make a vegetable soup.

- **Medicinal**

It is given to mentally disturbed children who suffer from hallucinations – for example imagining being chased. Herbalists, however, do not reveal how the medicine is made – part of the family heritage.

For coughs, cook the root and leaves and take 1 glass 3 times daily for 7 days.

Women in prolonged labour can also drink it as it eases child birth and relieves post partum pains and stress.

The liquid from its boiled leaves is good for dysentery. Dosage:1 glass 3 times a day for 7 days.

Goats with problems giving birth are given the leaves to eat.

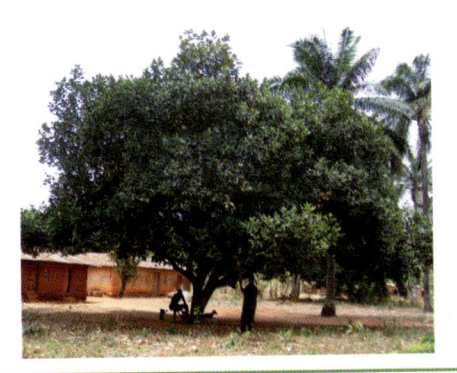

- **Cultural**

The tree serves as an idol (*Alijẹnu/Ẹbọ*).

Often planted in front of homes it is generally believed to prevent attack by witches.

Ọda makes excellent live fences also useful for the demarcation of graves.

- **Other uses**

As the picture shows, many compounds have this tree. Women in particular like to have it because the leaves make good vegetable soup and its prunings good firewood. As the tree becomes scarce in the wild, its use becomes less frequent in making mortar, pestles, furniture and firewood. Where still found women sell its leaves for medicine and soup.

Its sap, often used as gum, is considered particularly useful in fixing worn and torn bank notes.

Ọda improves soil fertility and provides an excellent shade. Its lack of a strong root makes it vulnerable during storms as it can be easily uprooted, resulting in damage to buildings.

Gmelina arborea
Igala: *Gmelina*
Common: Gmelina

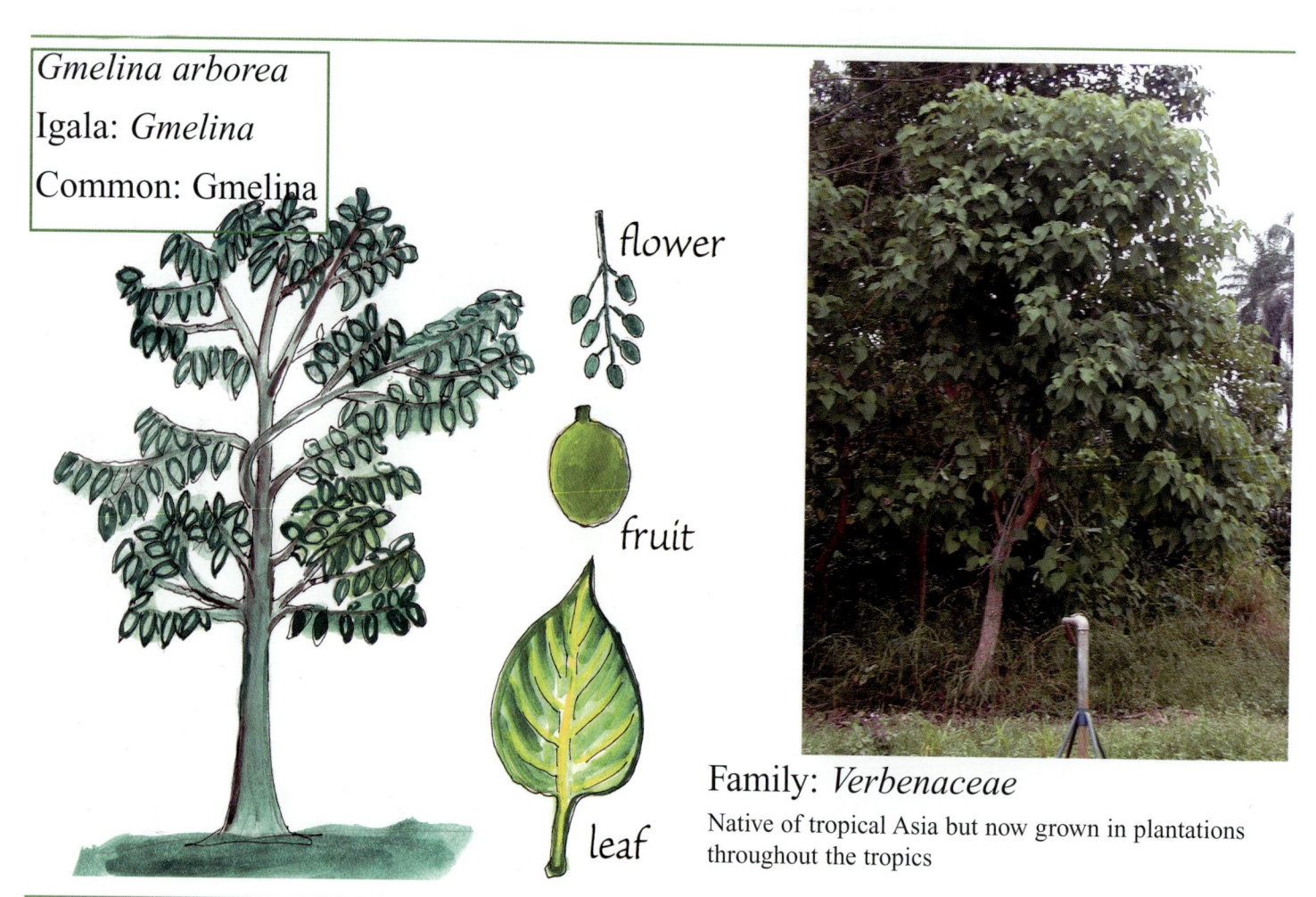

flower

fruit

leaf

Family: *Verbenaceae*
Native of tropical Asia but now grown in plantations throughout the tropics

•Food

Gmelina has no value as food.

•Medicinal

Perhaps surprisingly, considering it is a newcomer to the region, Gmelina is used frequently in medicinal formulations, usually in combination with either leaves, barks or the roots of other trees.

•Cultural

Gmelina had a limited presence here until the advent of a World Bank project known as the Ayangba Agricultural Development Project (AADP) in 1977.

Hitherto there were some government plantations of teak and gmelina but the AADP project made available 1 million seedlings of teak, gmelina and eucalyptus. These were distributed throughout the region. Although not all were planted, those who were wise enough to plant them do not regret their decision.

Teak and gmelina in particular are heading gradually towards the status of cash crops, just as eucalyptus definitely takes its place among the medicinal trees.

Gmelina has not as yet become part of traditional usage like the palms and iroko and other long established trees of the region. However, its acceptance shows people are not resistant to good things that contribute to their well-being.

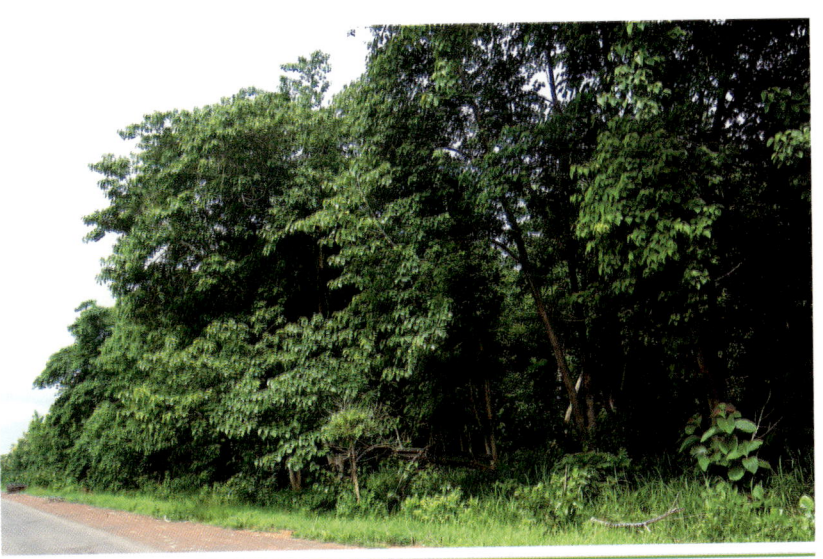

Gmelina plantation

•Other uses

This fast-growing tree makes excellent firewood, and other trees tend to be compared to it in this regard. It is very common to see stacks of Gmelina firewood for sale along the roadside, as can be seen in the photographs. Women earn much money from the sale of such wood.

Fast growing, Gmelina can be coppiced up to ten times, and cut for firewood in as little as two to three years after planting.

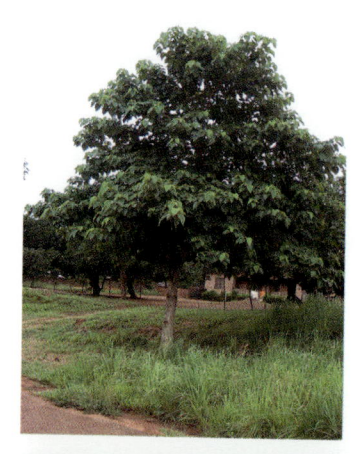

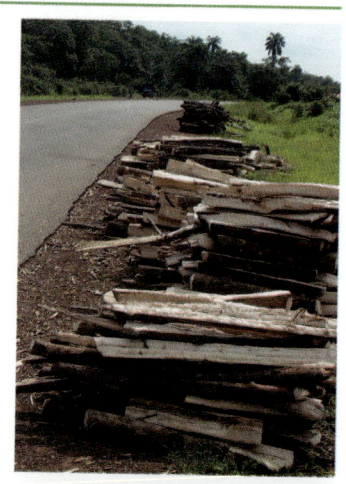

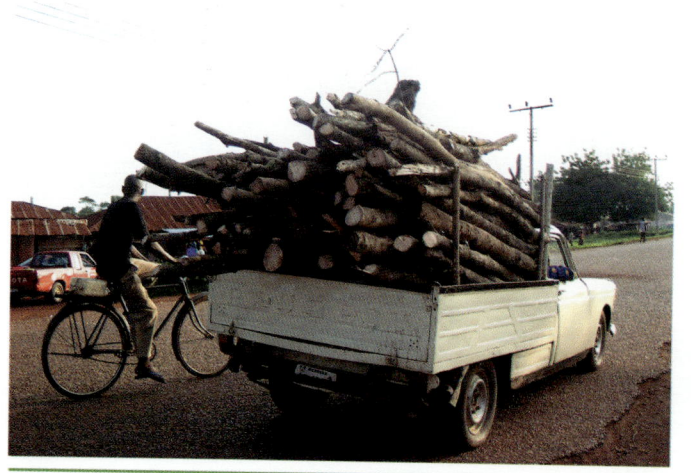

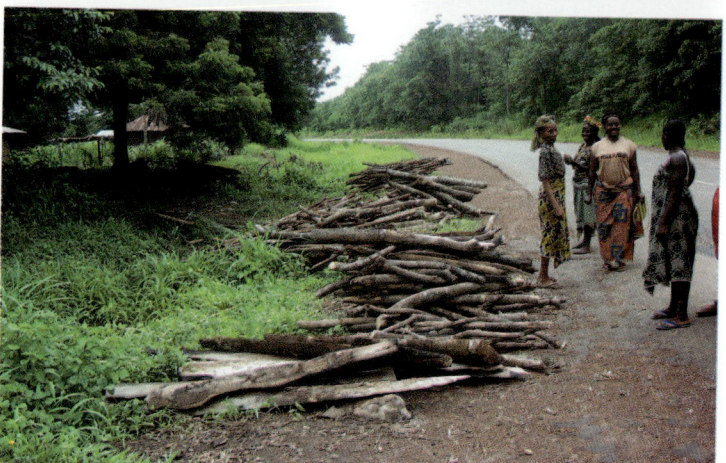

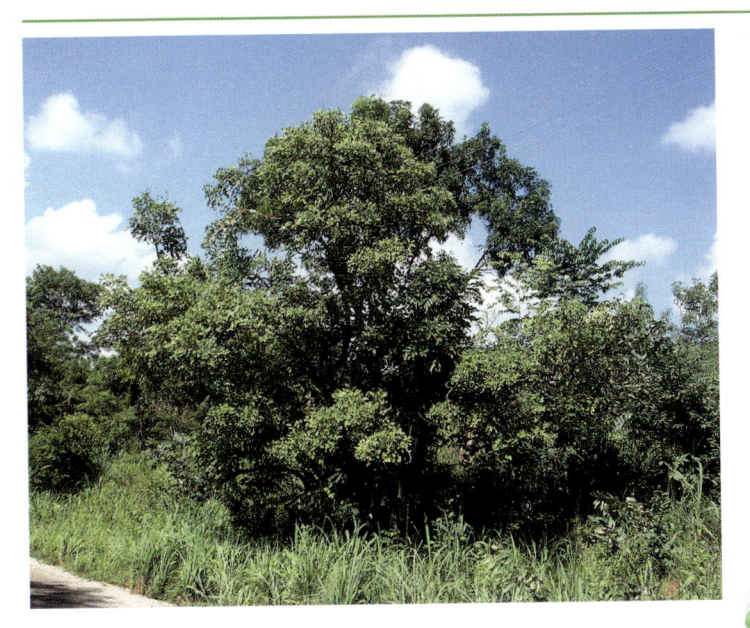

Hannoa undulata
Igala: *Odobala, Umopula*

Family: *Simaroubaceae*

A savannah tree with grey corky bark that is deeply furrowed. Flowers are yellow-cream in colour and sweetly scented. When ripe the fruits are black.

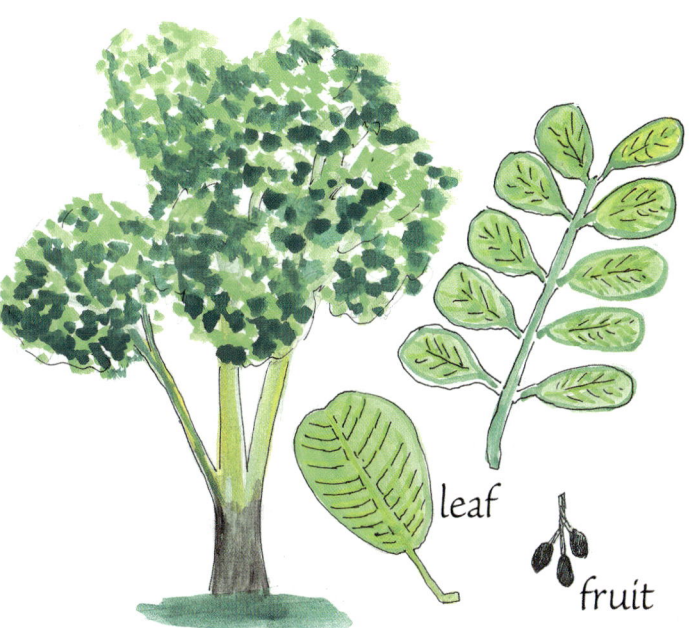

leaf

fruit

75

•Food

The fruits are edible.

•Medicinal

The leaf is boiled and a glass of the liquid is taken 3 times daily for stomach ache and malaria fever.

•Cultural

A special seat for women is made from its wood selling in large numbers within the region.

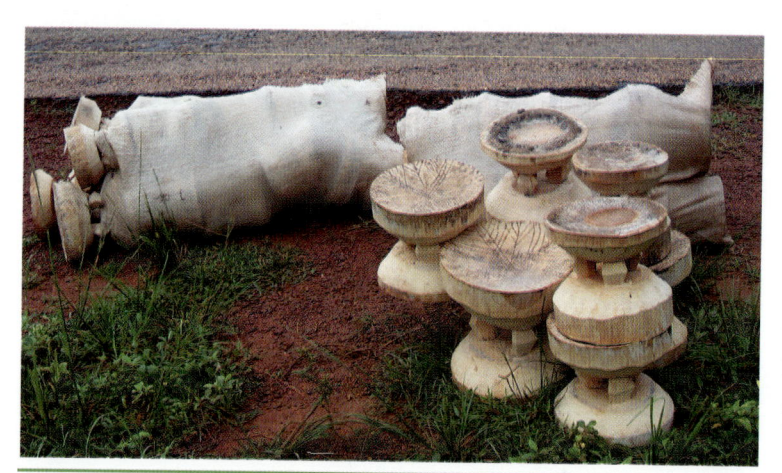

The wood is also used to make a local game

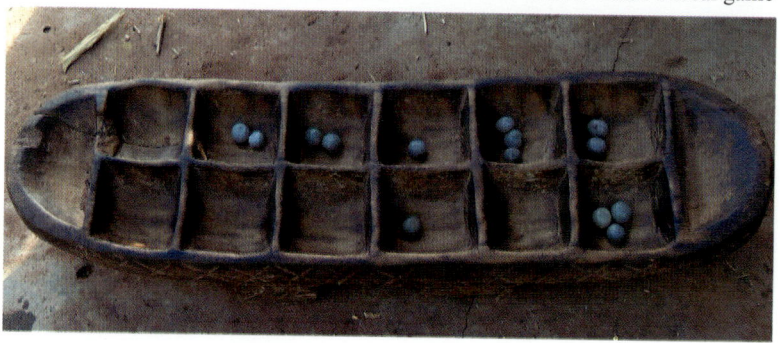

•Other uses

Good for firewood but no longer available in most places.

It was often used for domestic and office furniture but its now almost impossible to find planks.

Handles for farm implements are highly valuable, but scarce.

The tree which is a big loss for the flora of Igala and Bassa has not been replaced.

If leaves are available they are sold for medicine.

Leaf fall improves soil fertility.

Hymenocardia acida
Igala: *Ẹnache*
Common: Miombo Red-heart

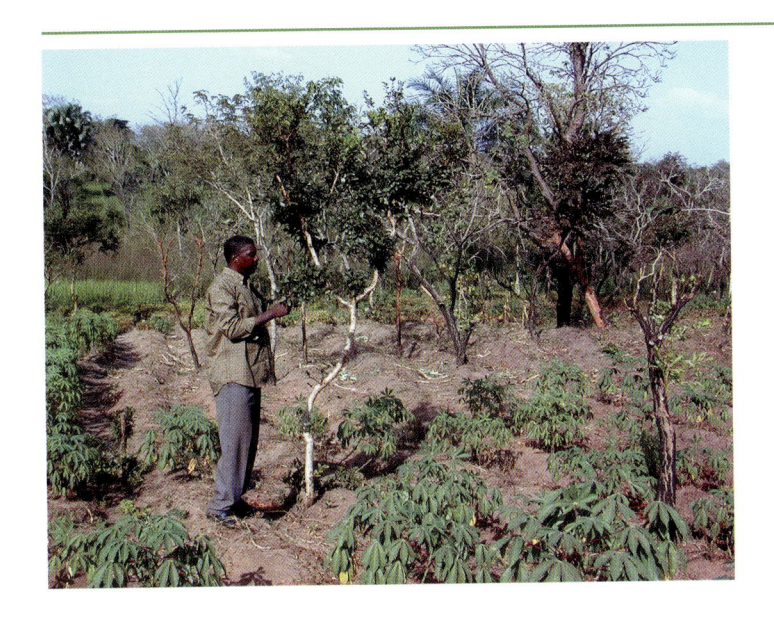

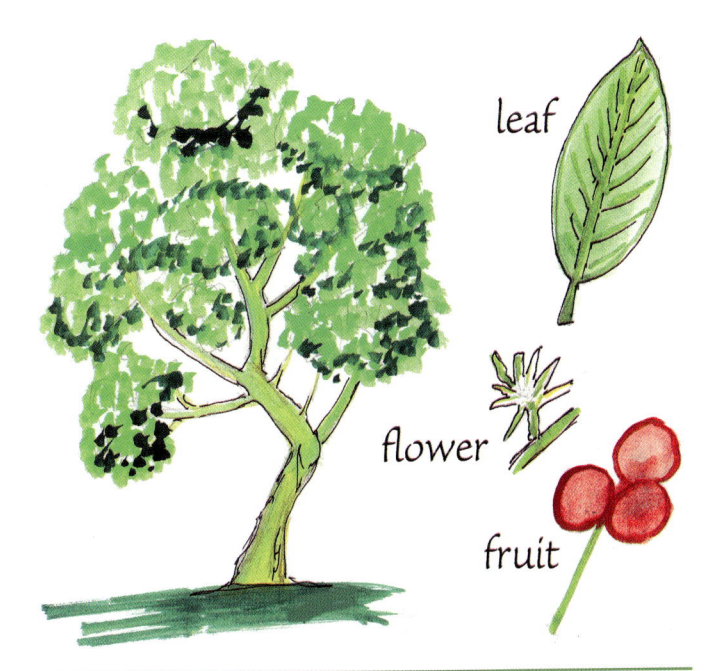

Family: *Euphorbiaceae*

A savannah shrub or small tree growing up to 20 ft tall

leaf

flower

fruit

•Food

No value as food.

•Cultural

No cultural value.

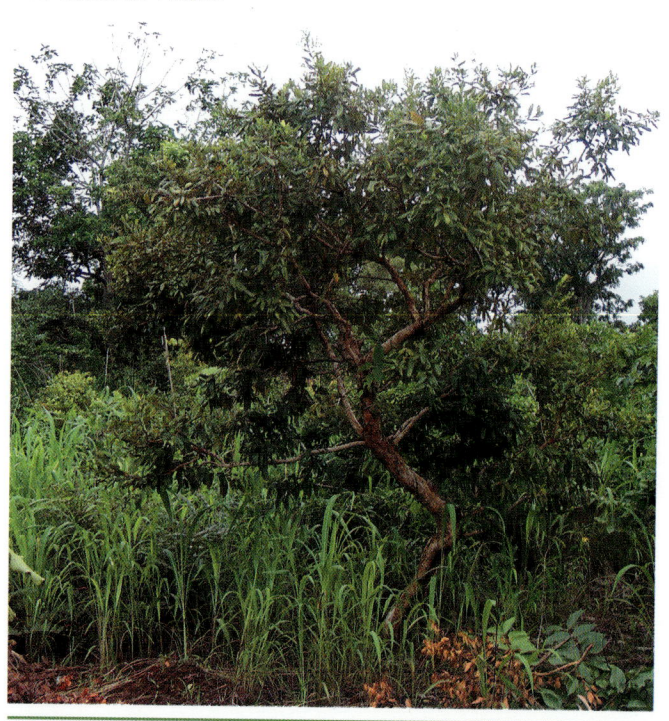

•Medicinal

Its flaky bark can be wrung to make a powder used to cure aching loins and skin diseases such as ringworm.

Ẹnache leaves, roots and bark are combined with *itado* stem and boiled for treating asthma, TB and coughs. Dosage: 1 glass taken 3 times daily for 7 days.

To cure dysentery and stomach ache its leaves are boiled. Dosage: 1 glass taken 3 times daily for 7 days.

Pregnant women also take this medicine 4 months before delivery, usually 3 times daily.

This same medicine also cures malaria – one glass 3 times daily for 7 days.

Pneumonia (*adakpo* or *oma imiabia*) common in children can be cured if *ẹnache* leaves and bark are boiled and the liquid divided. Part is reserved for the child's bath, the rest administered orally. Dosage: half a glass 3 times daily for 7 days.

Ẹnache: Iji Ọbiẹkoli majotule. The best leading fuel wood.

•Other uses

Once regarded as one of the best firewoods in the region, it is now endangered and therefore a luxury. However, it can still be found in small quantities as shown in the picture. It does not absorb rain, so housewives can use it even if they forget to bring it indoors.

Though the fork stick is slender, it is strong enough to make a catapult handle.

Like ompanions, granaries, local beds, local parlours (*atakpa*), hoe and cutlass handles are made with it.

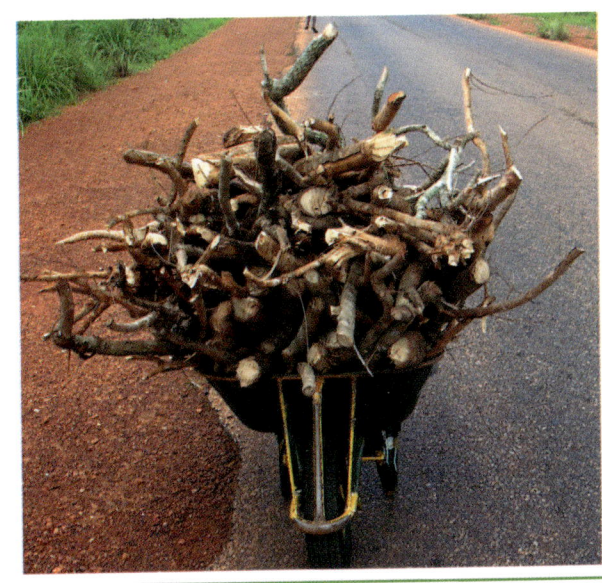

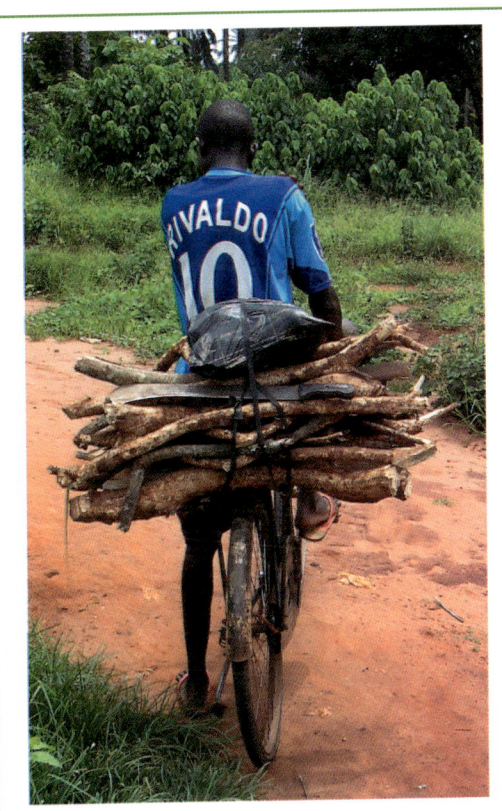

Frames from *Ɛnache* are plastered with clay for local houses.

Women market its leaves and roots for medicinal purposes.

Farmers use it for yam staking.

It produces massive quantities of leaves used as biomass.

As it is now endangered, goats no longer have access to it.

Irvingia gabonensis

Igala: *Ọrọ-Egili, Ọrọ-Egiri*

Common: Bush Mango

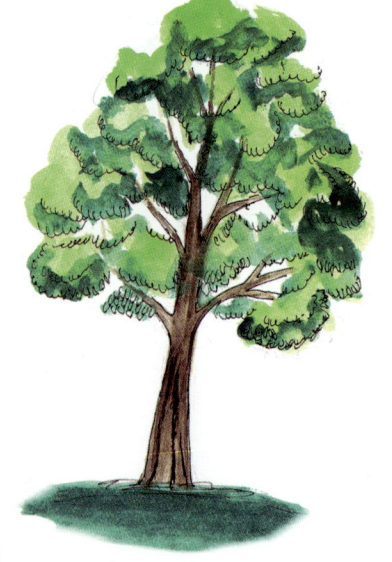

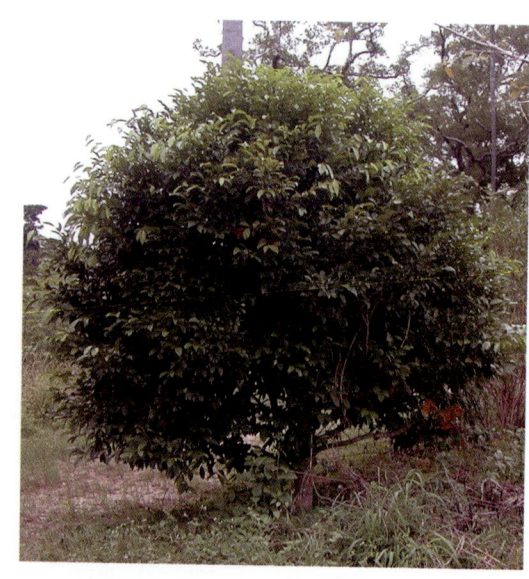

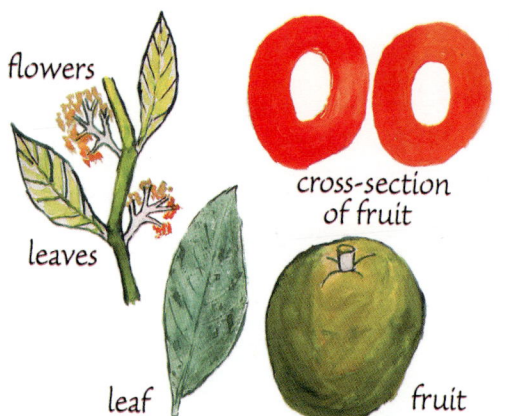

Family: *Irvingiaceae*

A forest tree growing up to 120 ft tall with dark green shiny foliage. Flowers are fragrant and fruits are yellow-green. Often seen in or near towns and villages.

•Food

Bush mango fruits and nuts are edible; its seeds are an important ingredient in 'draw' soups.

Bush mango must not be confused with the popular mango fruit though the two fruits look alike.

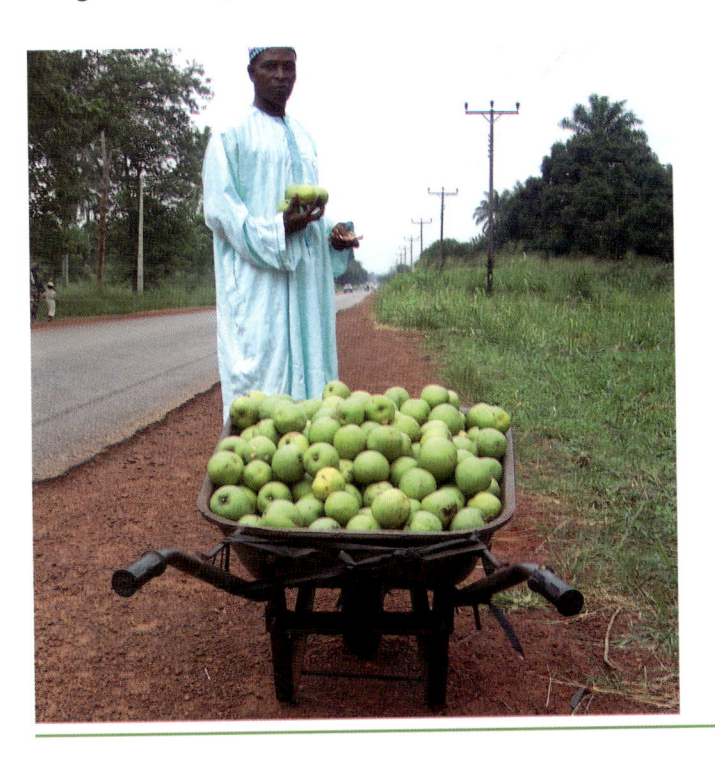

•Cultural

During annual festivals, its seeds become a most valuable ingredient for the preparation of draw soup. However, the low drawing capacity of *Irvingia gabonensis* soup as well as its bitter taste can devalue it somewhat if compared to *Irvingia wombulu*. Both of these Ọrọ trees are now endangered and less common, and because of that attitudes are changing.

•Medicinal

The leaves and bark of the bush mango are boiled and the liquid used to treat fever, dysentery and measles.

To cure catarrh in a newborn baby, the bark is boiled in water over a fire made from bush mango wood. Some water is reserved for bathing the baby. A spoonful is given to the baby twice daily for 7 days. After this the mixture can be renewed.

The bark often used as a chewing stick because is also believed to cure toothache.

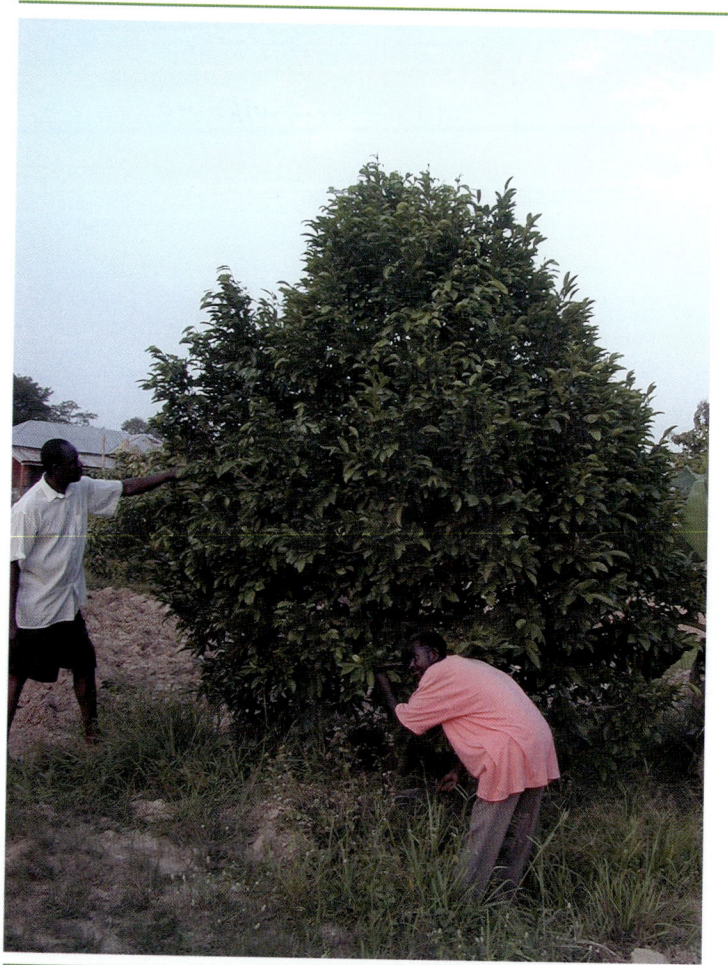

•Other uses

The bush mango is highly valued in the region.

Its wood is only rarely used for firewood except when for example a tree has been uprooted by a storm or branches are left after pruning.

A bush mango tree can be sawn into planks used in the construction of local furniture, granaries, local parlours and shelter in the farm or compound.

Like its sister the okra tree, its green leaves ensure soil fertility through the biomass produced and the nitrogen fixed.

The picture shows the tree at the early stages of growth. It has produced fruit at this level of development.

Family: *Irvingiaceae*

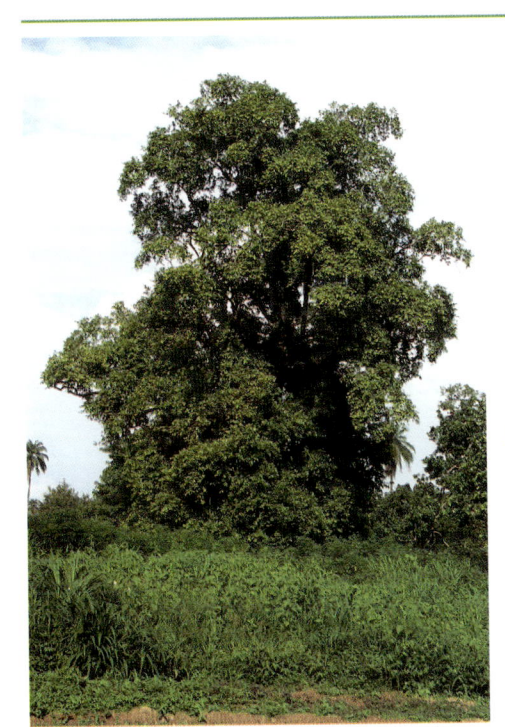

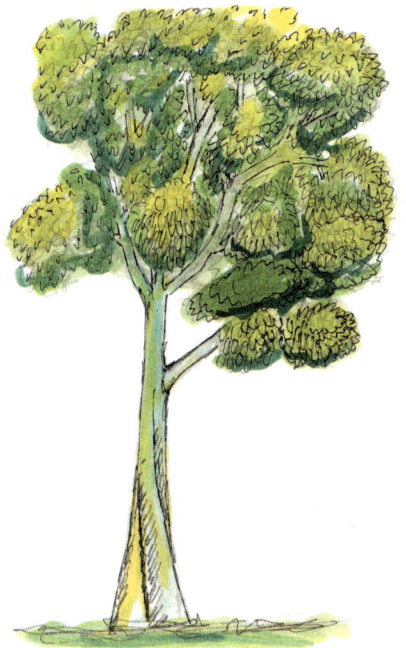

Irvingia wombulu
Igala: Ọrọ-Ayikpẹlẹ
Common: Okra tree

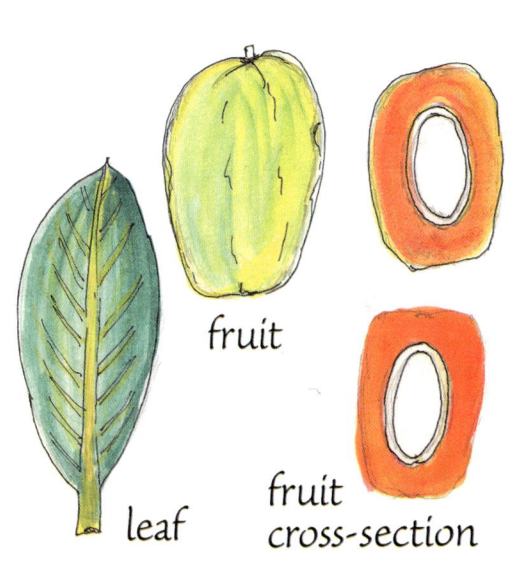

leaf

fruit

fruit cross-section

•Food

The fruits are much enjoyed and the seeds used for making soup.

•Cultural

The seed is an important ingredient for 'draw' soup prepared on the first day of festivals, especially the annual ones during which sacrifice is made to the ancestors. Only visitors enjoy this specialist dish as the ancestors feast on yam with *egusi* melon soup.

> *Ogbodaga : Ifa ibi kimanẹhi:*
> If the oracle turns upside down in the course of consultation, it forebodes real problems,
> death or sickness.

•Medicinal

Its boiled leaves are used for stomach-ache and measles. A glass full of the warmed liquid is taken 3 times a day for 7 days. It can be renewed if necessary.

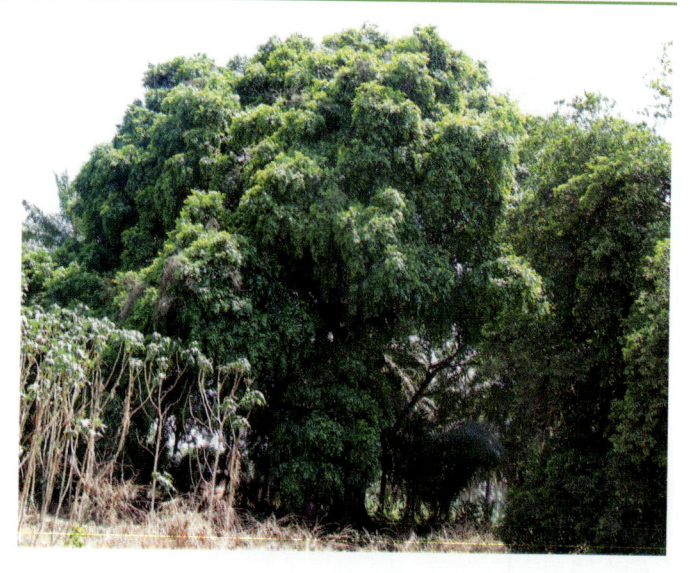

•Other uses

Respected as an excellent firewood but it is only used when it dies. Prunings are also good for firewood.

Ideal for handles of hoes, cutlasses and axes but rarely used nowadays as the wood is valued too highly.

A top class cash crop with much income derived from the sale of fruit, seed and leaves

It has a long-standing reputation as a fertilizer tree.

Khaya senegalensis
Igala: *Ago*
Common: Mahogany

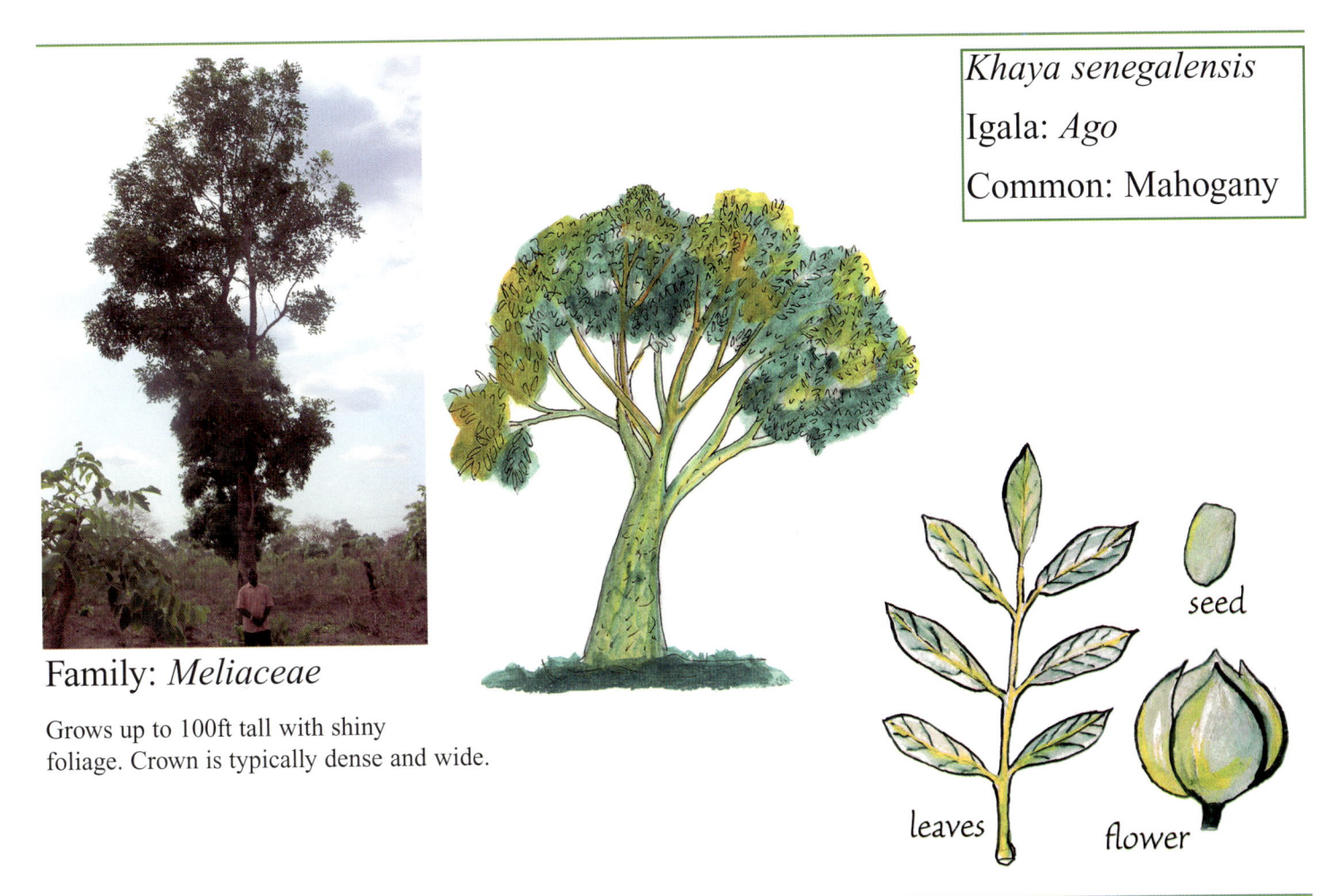

Family: *Meliaceae*

Grows up to 100ft tall with shiny foliage. Crown is typically dense and wide.

leaves

seed

flower

85

•Food

No value as food.

•Cultural

Traditional believers worship beneath it. The artifacts associated with this worship are everywhere to be seen, most of the images carved out of its wood represent local deities.

The images from this wood, locally known as *Eyicha*, are in great demand for the funerals of traditional believers. All the children, including grandchildren, come with these images, accompanied by a masquerade and music to celebrate transition to the ancestors.

•Medicinal

To cure typhoid the bark is soaked in cold water and 1 glass taken 3 times daily for 7 days. If after 1 week the patient is still suffering, repeat the dosage from a freshly made batch.

To treat malaria fever and anaemia, boil bark and leaves. Take the warmed liquid 3 times daily for 1 week and the ailment will go.

To cure oedema, grind some of the bark into paste. Cook the remainder and wash the body with warm liquid and then apply the paste to the affected part after washing well with the water.

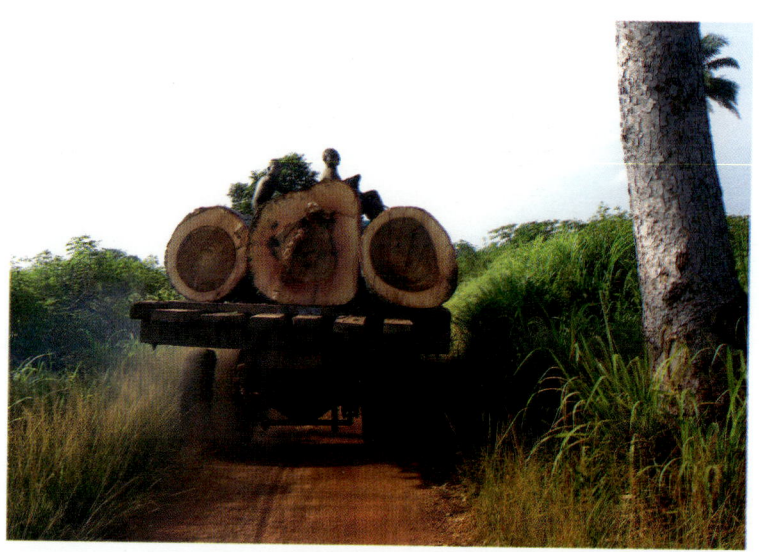

The first leg of the export trail – cutting of trees.

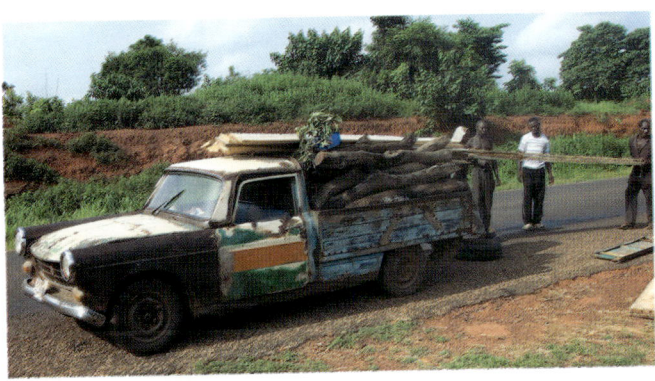

•Other uses

Like all good hardwoods, mahogany is now listed amongst the endangered tree species as there is practically no replanting. This has an impoverishing effect on the region as the wood is sold as planks for export and very few trees replanted.

Mahogany is excellent for firewood, though it is rarely used nowadays because of high cost. Domestic and office furniture, frames of houses, granaries and local parlours (*atapka*) are also rarely made from it due to its high cost.

The Mahogany tree provides protection from the sun for humans and animals alike, especially during the dry season. Beneath its shade, farm produce is threshed, food pounded and children play games whilst adults take a well deserved rest from the toils of the day.

Its dried wood is used for pit toilets.

It also offers a beauty which is restful and inspiring, and providing a quiet spot where children do their homework.

In the pictures the trunks being delivered to a compound will be used as building materials.

Women sell its bark, fruit and leaves mainly for medicinal purposes.

A local mahogany seat generates valuable income.

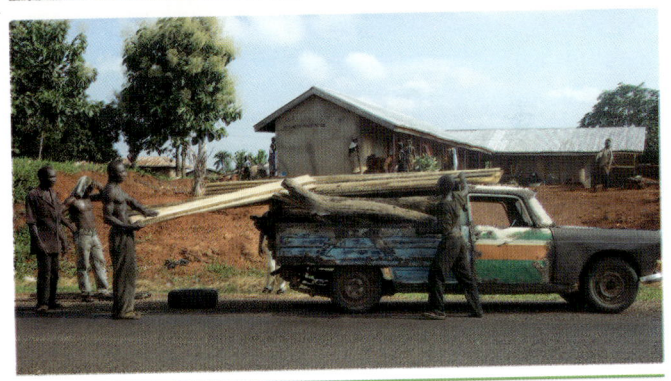

•Other uses

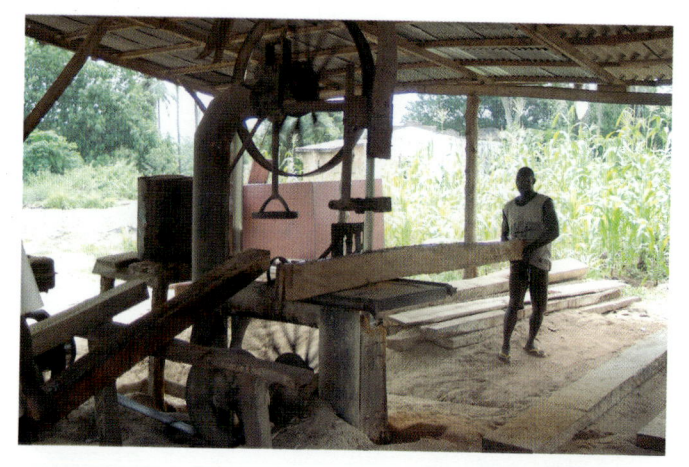

Mortars and pestles, hoe, cutlass and axe handles are a good source of income for the producers.

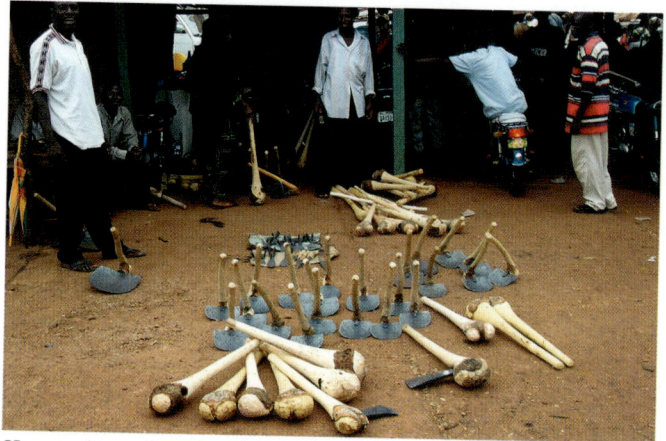

Cutting of the trunks into planks (Egume Sawmill).

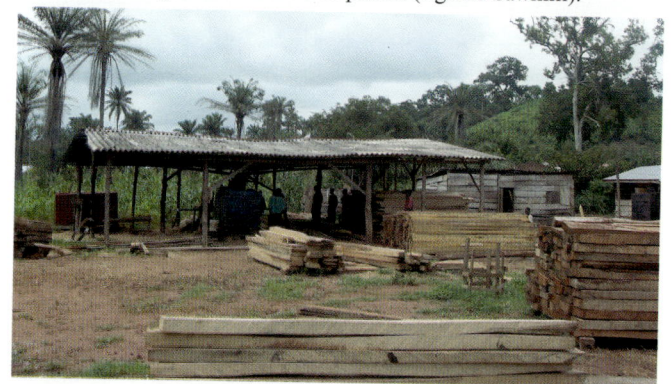

Hoes and axes for sale, Idah market.

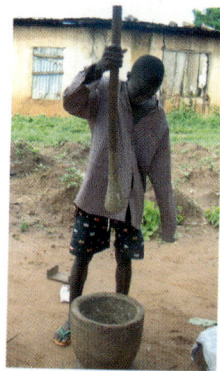

Using a mortar and pestle made from mahogany.

Kigelia africana

Igala: *Ẹbiẹ, Unya*

Common: Sausage Tree

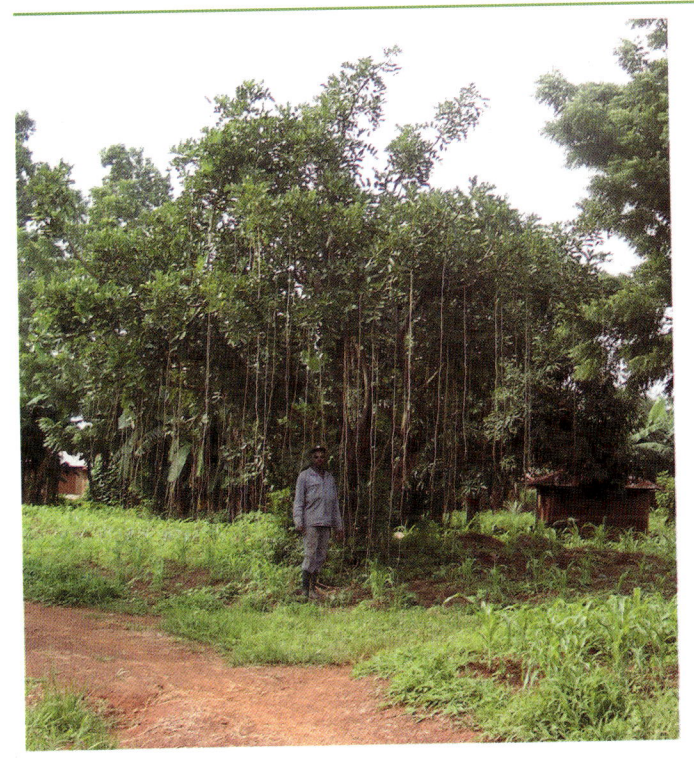

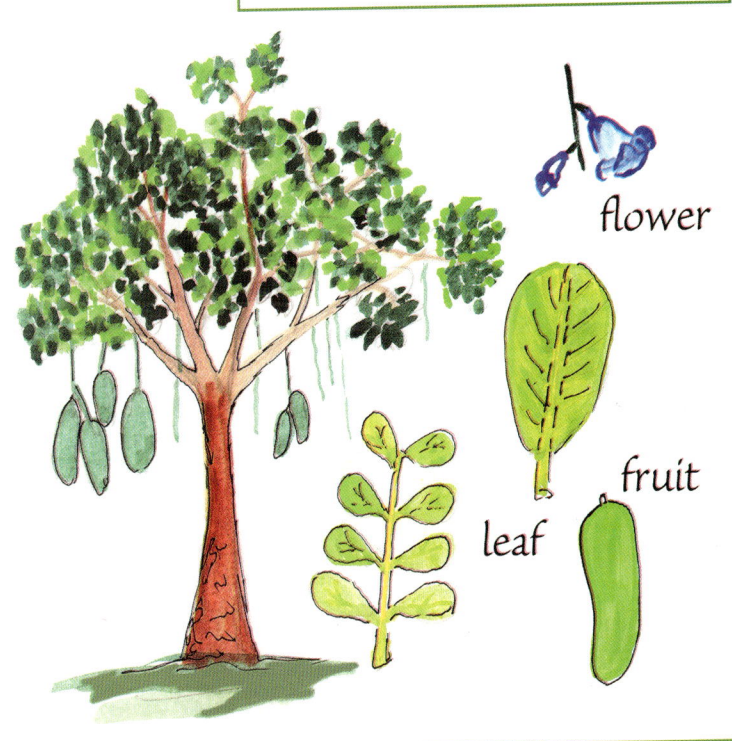

Family: *Bignoniaceae*

Tree growing up to 20 to 50 ft tall. Flowers variable in colour (red to yellow to blue to green). Fruits are like long sausages, hence the English name.

•Food

No value as food.

•Cultural

To prevent theft, its fruit is placed on top of properties; anyone who removes property thus guarded will have a sickness known as *Ębię* (a form of oedema) for punishment.

If not treated on time an open wound appears which can lead to death. As a precaution in forestalling death, offenders have to confess their crime before treatment can commence. It is recommended that such a confession be made in the presence of the fruit.

This is an anecdote told by Egbunu Acholo (herbalist) about the *Ębię*:

Oga-ębię kimanę ifa ębo

When the sickness comes (as a result of stealing), there is no point in consulting the oracle. Every one knows your problem. Only very rare cases can be treated.

When coming to remove your belongings you must tell the *Ębię* in a loud voice you are returning to claim your goods. People are advised to wear the same clothes when returning for their goods as when they first placed the fruit onto them.

To treat the wound, boil the bark and leaf together to provide the liquid for washing the wound. A paste is made from the bark only and applied after washing with the water. The treatment is administered externally.

Oga-ębię kimanę-ogwu.

Sickness from this source has no cure other than that provided by the herbalist. So bad is this sickness, it can affect your unborn children. The penalty is therefore 'hereditary'.

•Medicinal

To cure oedema part of its bark is ground into a paste and the rest boiled. The warm liquid is used to wash the body and then the paste applied.

This same formula and method of application is used to treat swollen breasts after childbirth.

Ẹbiẹ leaves boiled with a tender teak leaf are used to cure anaemia. One glass is taken 3 times a day for 7 days. This same dosage will also help with many children's diseases. Children often can't explain their illness so this is a good remedy to test the severity of an illness.

The same formulation eases the pangs of childbirth if a glass is taken 3 times daily from the fourth month of pregnancy. To reduce oedema during pregnancy a woman applies a paste made from the bark of *Ẹbiẹ* and *baobab* before going to bed.

•Other uses

As it absorbs moisture easily, it is used for firewood only in an emergency. Firewood determines the taste of the food and is therefore important in cooking.

People do not enjoy its shade while in fruit because a falling fruit could cause death. Outside the fruiting season there is shade for all.

Its bark and leaves are the main source of income.

Biomass from the tree helps maintain soil fertility.

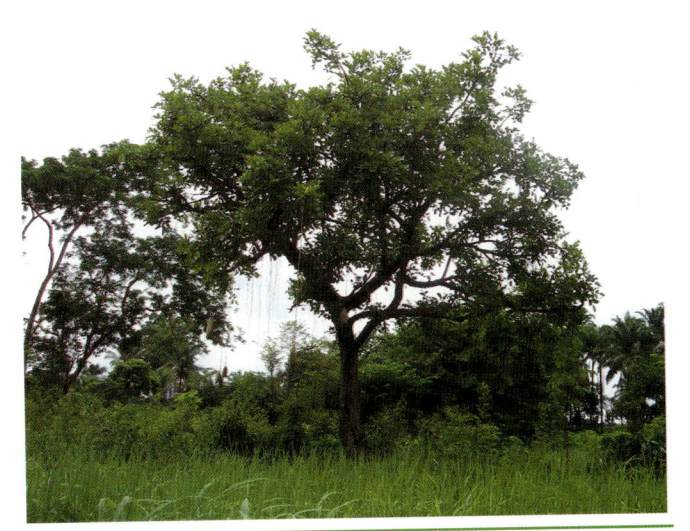

Landolphia amoena
Igala: *Abo*

leaf

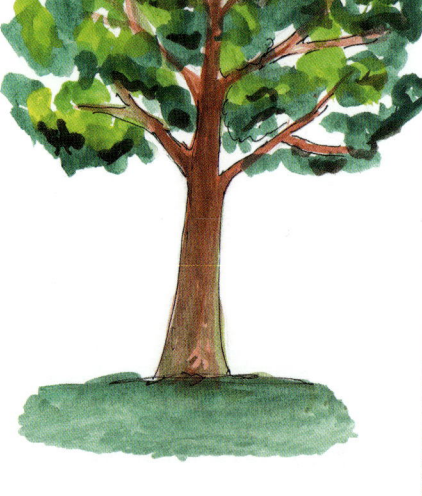

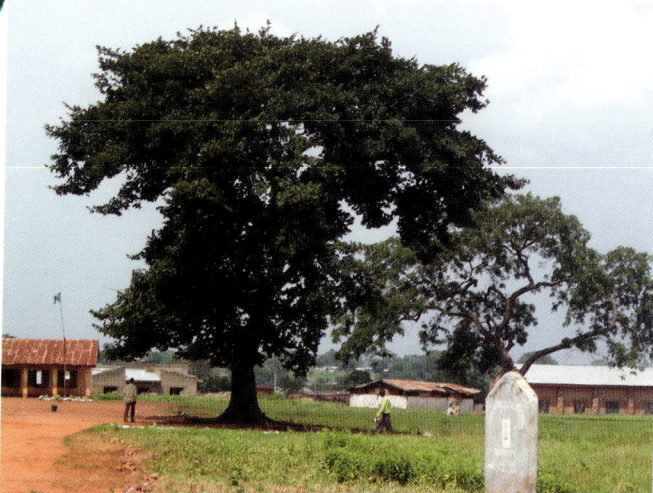

Family: *Apocynaceae*

•Food

The mushroom is tasty and adds to the dish in the same way fish does. Protein is rare in the diet so this supplement is highly valued.

The adage goes as follows: If the slave (*adu*) is deprived of eating fish, no one can stop him eating mushroom. A thought for the day!

Adu majeja yajoru.

•Cultural

Artists use *abo* wood to carve their idols

Instruments for masquerade head are manufactured locally using *abo*.

•Medicinal

To cure snakebite grind *abo* and *uloko* roots and the head of a dead snake to a paste and apply to the affected area. Part of the paste is mixed with palm wine or water and 1 glass taken twice daily for 2 weeks.

For women suffering from stomach ache, *abo* is ground with *uloko* and *ochimichi* roots. Warm water is added and taken 1 glass 3 times a day for 30 days.

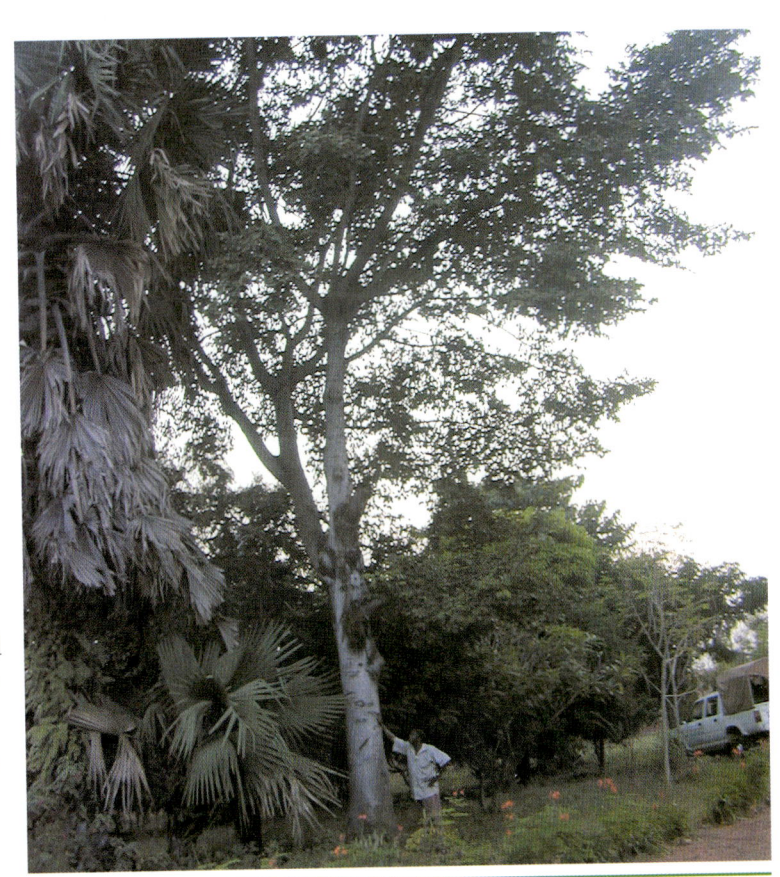

•Other uses

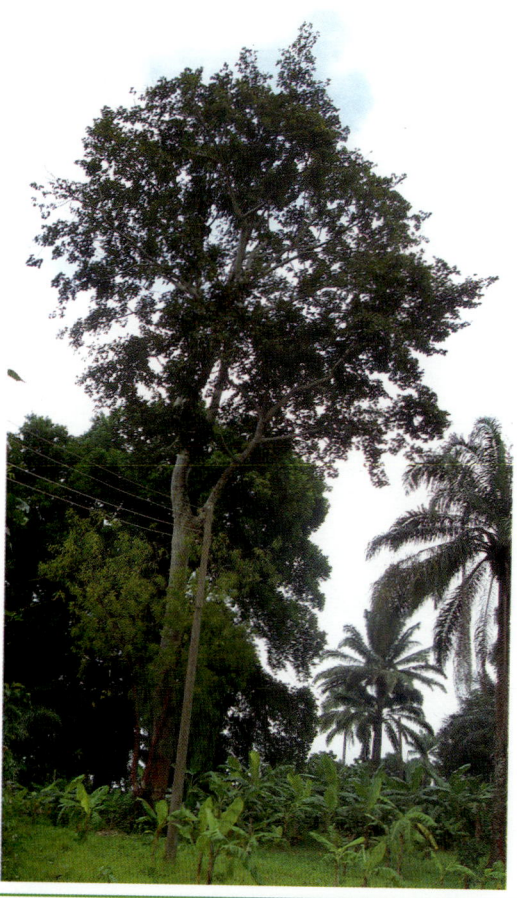

It always has foliage and provides a regular supply of nutrients to the surrounding soil.

What more can this picture say? – Rich soil and good maize.

Abo enjoys new status in the firewood category as 'it burns like gmelina'.

Traditionally it has been used for domestic and office furniture, handles for hoes, cutlasses and axes.

It provides building materials, especially frames to which clay is applied, particularly useful for *atakpas* and granaries.

In its early stages it produces shade, but as it develops shade decreases.

A good provider of fodder despite its height; goats in particular like it.

Considered ornate, it helps develop an aesthetical sense where such resources are appreciated.

Profit is derived from its timber sales.

Mushroom growing beneath it fetches high prices in the market. 'Sold in the market like fish' means it is used to prepare soup.

Lannea nigritana

Igala: *Echikala, Igogo*

Common: Hog Plum

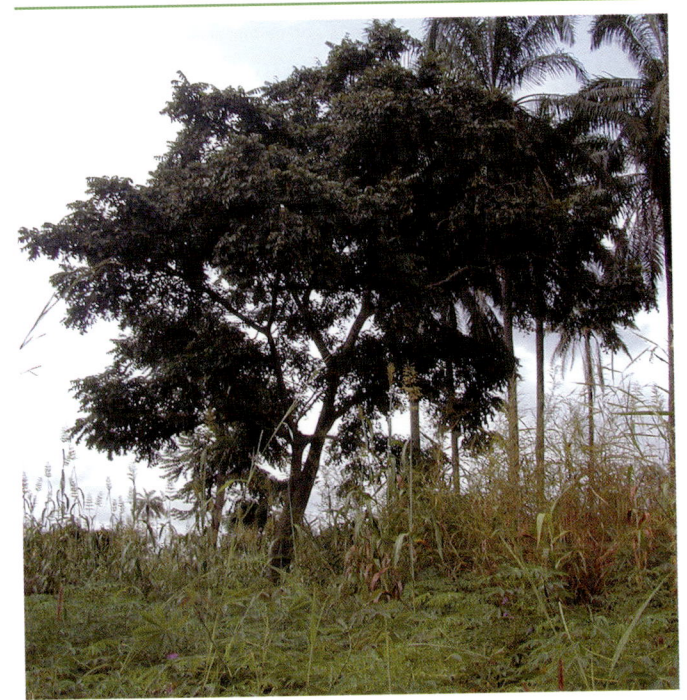

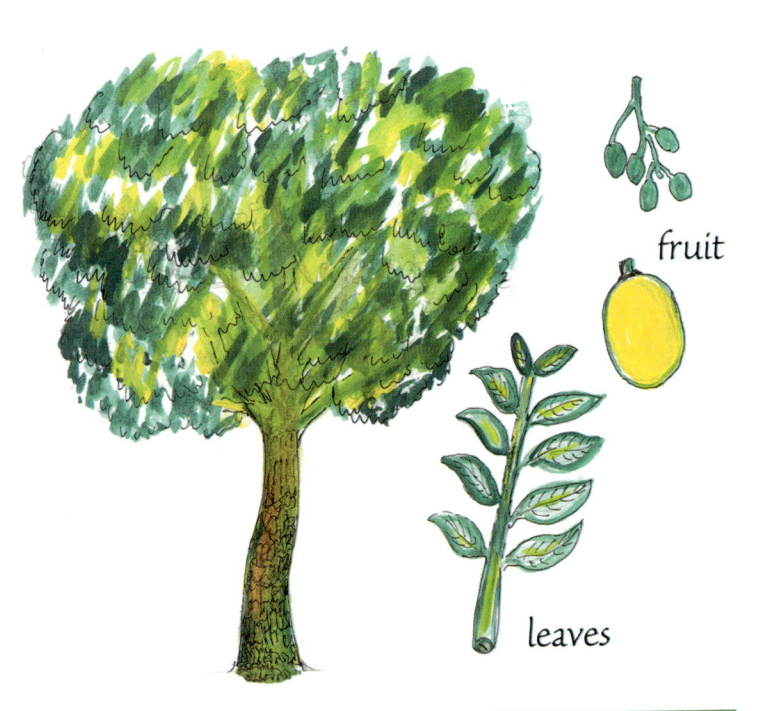

Family: *Anacardiaceae*

Grows up to 45 ft with wide and sparse branching. The flowers are yellow and produced when leafless. When fully ripe the fruit is black. Occurs in the drier parts of forest regions.

fruit

leaves

•Food

Its fruit is edible, but too many plums damage teeth which temporarily reduces capacity for chewing.

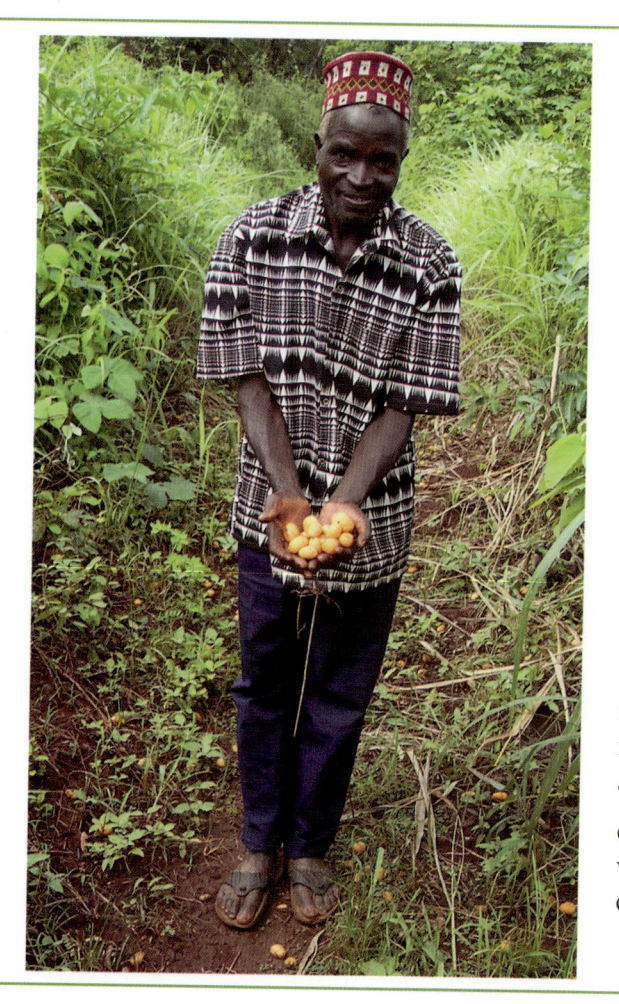

•Cultural

Like the *ogichi* its major use is to provide a clear indication as to where graves are located and to mark boundaries between plots.

With the use of hog plum leaves, a special exercise is traditionally performed to help identify thieves. Without them such a ceremony is considered invalid.

The wood is also suitable for making local traps.

•Medicinal

Good for the treatment of stomach disorders after child-birth. The leaf is squeezed in water, filtered and then given to the mother. There is no specific measurement. This drink also helps release a retained placenta.

The leaf and skin are recommended for breast cancer. Boil leaves and bark, and press the hot water to the breast twice daily with a face cloth for 14 days.

The liquid from the boiled bark and leaves cures tooth ache, malaria fever and stomach pain. The dosage is 1 glass 3 times a day for 7 days.

To cure toothache hold the liquid in your mouth for some time before swallowing it.

Leaves are given to goats before and after delivery to ease pain.

Leaf and fruit are sold in the market as medicine. Demand is high and the price good.

Health warning:

There are two types of hog plum. One of them is extremely poisonous. This is called *echikala-ukpewo* (the hog plum that kills goats). Consult your herbalist to ensure you do not confuse the two trees.

•Other uses

Well-liked as firewood despite its propensity to absorb water. It breaks easily, lights quickly, and reduces the burden of coaxing a fire to start.

As a white wood susceptible to woodworm, the timber is not the best for furniture .

Propagated easily and cheaply from cuttings, it is used for the construction of yam barns and granaries. However it is not suitable for traditional house building as a live fence would be destructive to a permanent structure.

Hog plum is traditionally used for the construction of a local seat which is popular with Igala masquerades (*akpa*).

Commonly used for pestle and canoe paddles, hoe and cutlass handles.

It has copious biomass, which degrades easily.

It provides moderate shade and doesn't grow too tall.

The tree is pretty but the stem is rough.

Goats eat its leaves.

Lophira laneolata

Igala: *Okopi*

Common: Iron tree

leaf

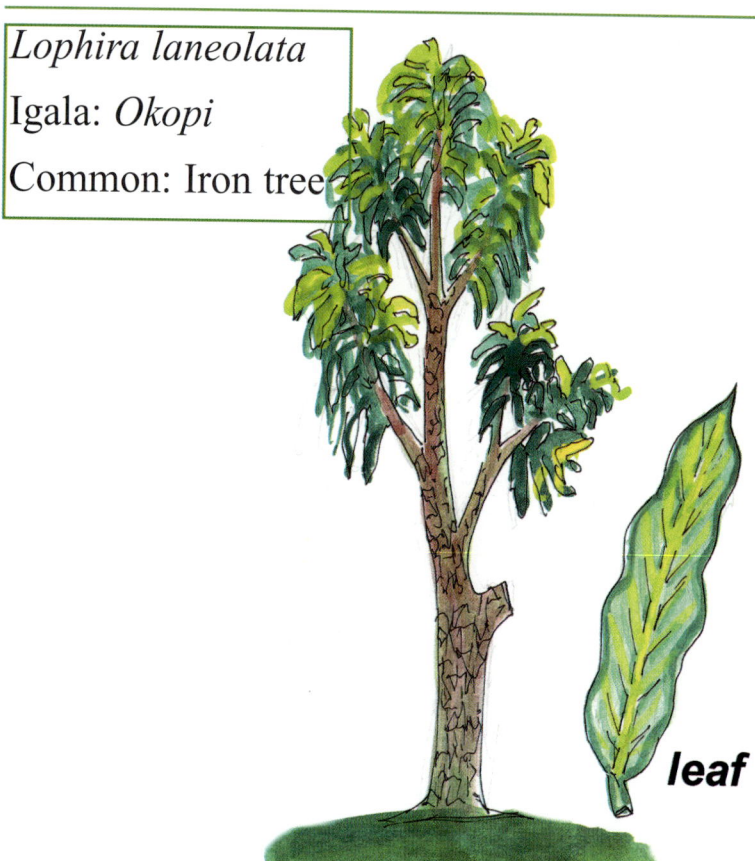

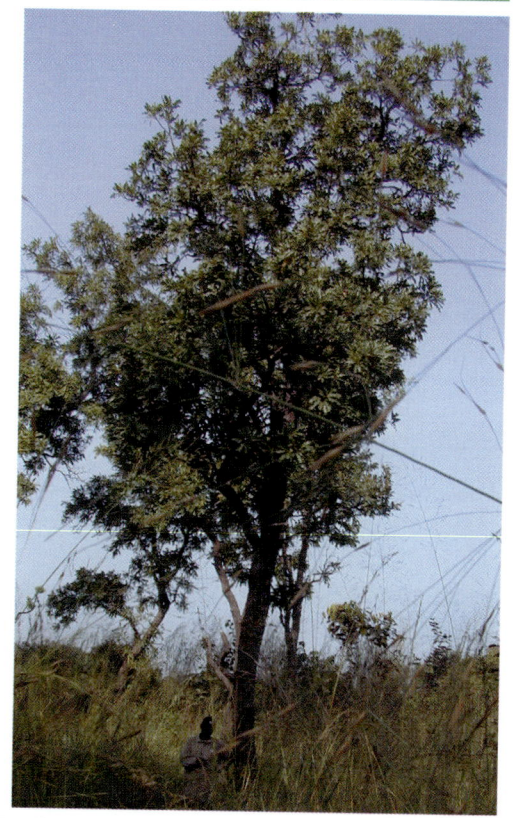

Family: *Ochnaceae*

A savannah tree growing up to 40 ft high. Trunk is usually rough and gnarled. Flowers are white.

•Food

It is not edible

•Cultural

Its leaves are placed on property left on the farm to protect it from thieves.

Any one venturing to steal goods thus protected will suffer from severe oedema and, should this be fatal, the victim will be buried in the bush without being accorded traditional rites.

•Medicinal

Mothers lacking breast milk boil its leaves with *ugbakolo* leaves and take 1 glass 3 times daily for 7 days.

Cough and fevers are relieved if its leaves are boiled with *ijili* leaves. One glass is taken 3 times daily for 7 days.

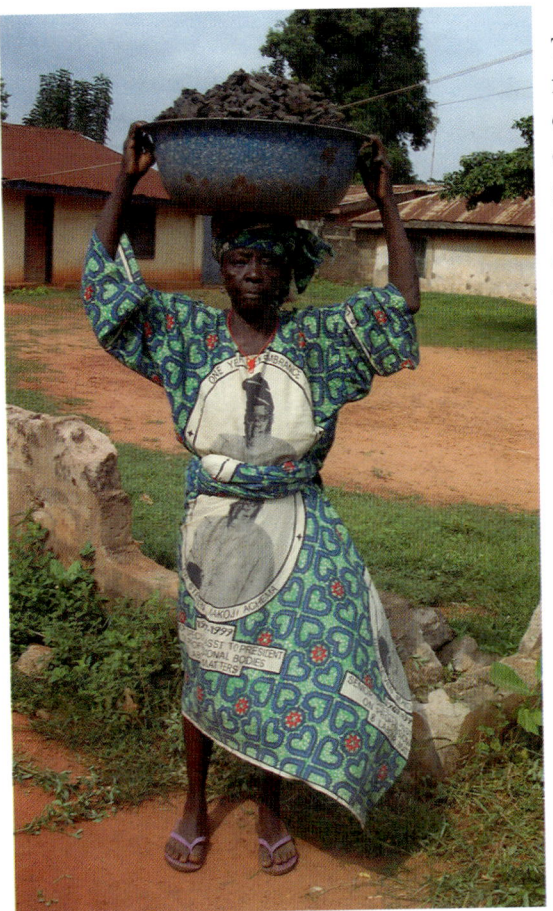

The bark is used for the treatment of headache and oedema. It is ground to a paste and applied externally 3 times a day for 7 days.

In the instance of severe oedema, when the body turns yellow, a paste made from a combination of *okopi* and *ogile* barks is applied externally twice daily for 7 days.

•Other uses

Good for firewood but not used frequently as it is endangered in some parts of the region.

Blacksmiths use it for charcoal because of its durability. It must be still abundant between Idah and Anyigba as sacks of charcoal are arranged here for sale and export to other parts of the country.

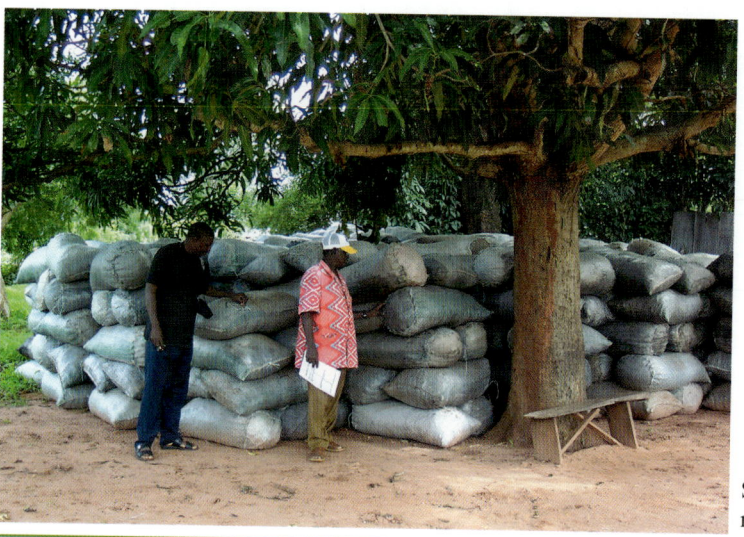

A hard wood suitable for making all types of furniture (seats tables, doors, beds and chairs) as it has resistance to woodworm. Furniture made from it provides a good source of income for carpenters who can afford to buy it.

The tree is good for the construction of canoes and paddles famous for their durability. However, they sink immediately if they capsize.

Both its fork stick and branches are used for building local houses, granaries, yam stores and *atakpas*. Pillars for local verandahs are made from it.

This tree is important in terms of land tenure in Igalaland. A tenant has to seek permission to plant it.

Its leaves and bark are sold in the market for medicinal use.

Children and some married women who are destitute sell the branches for firewood.

Sacks of charcoal by the road ready for export to the north of Nigeria.

Mangifera indica
Igala: *Umagolo*
Common: Mango

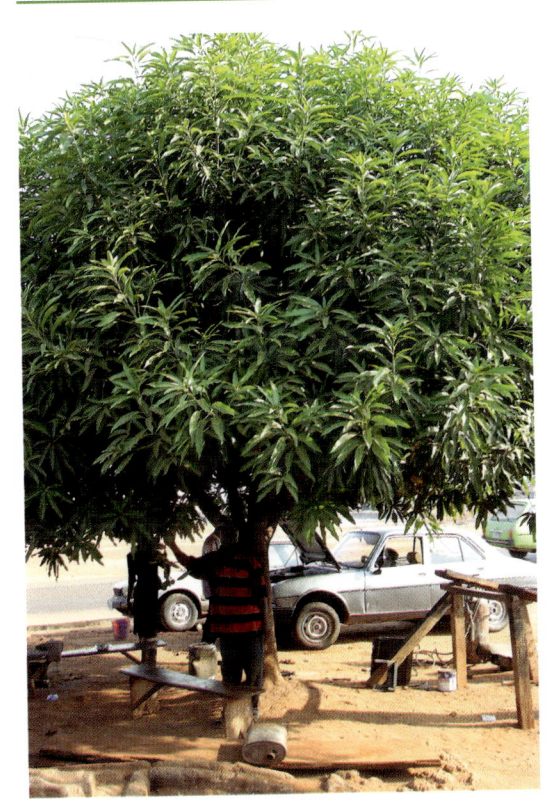

Family: *Anacardiaceae*

A native of India and now grown throughout the tropics. Widely cultivated, but also grows wild.

flower

flower stalk

leaf

fruit

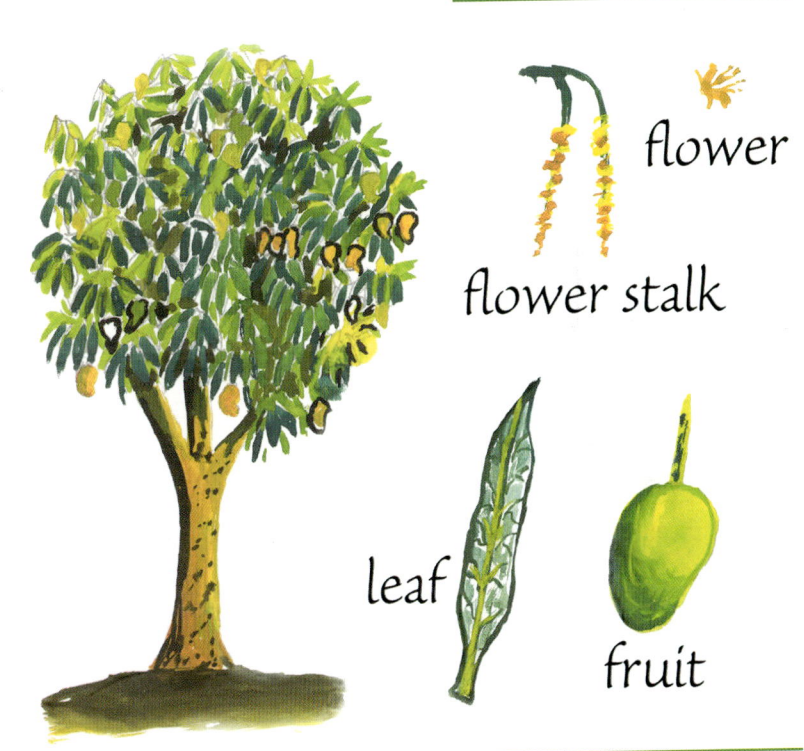

•Food

The mango is as welcome as a shower of rain when it ripens in February or March, as at this time food supplies are at their lowest and heat at its highest.

Everyone regards the refreshing mango fruit as a gift. There would be little to eat during the pre planting period (February to June) were it not for mangoes and cashew (whose fruits ripen prior to that of mango). Numerous improved varieties of mango have been bred in the last decade, further enhancing its palatability.

A sweet fruit, children love it as a snack at break time. Petty traders sell it outside every school.

A local juice known as *Mendi* is now being made from mango in the Ankpa area with pepper and *alu* added. Although not yet commercialized, it is being used socially in the same way as local cereal drinks such as *obiolo* (a non-alcoholic drink made from guinea corn and maize). This is a welcome initiative as millions of mangoes are wasted each year.

It propagates easily and requires little maintenance.

•Cultural

Mango has no cultural value in the region.

•Medicinal

Used primarily for the treatment of malaria fever and stomach ache.

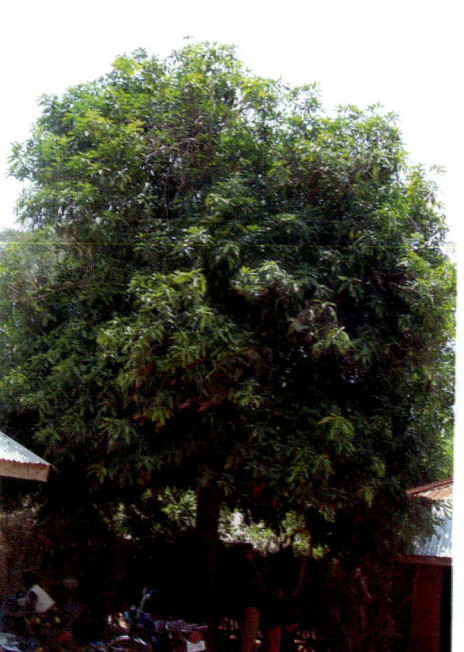

If there are symptoms of typhoid fever and jaundice, leaves of pawpaw, guava, African almond, and acacia are boiled together and 1 glass taken 3 times daily for 7 days.

For catarrh, add lemon grass leaves in the same dosage. To gain optimum advantage the head is covered with a cloth and held over the pot for as long as possible.

To cure anaemia, the bark is boiled with tender teak leaves and 1 glass taken 3 times a day for 7 days.

Mango also cures cough and pneumonia. Boil the bark and drink the liquid 3 times daily for 7 days.

To cure pneumonia, boil the bark and leaves and drink once after boiling. Use some of the remainder to wash the body twice daily for 7 days. The liquid has to be warmed each time.

•Other uses

Good for firewood, but now used only when cut down or pruned.

Mango wood is never used for furniture, although its forked sticks are for granaries, *atakpas* and for the handles of farm implements. Mango wood is not as durable as other hard woods.

Although mango leaves do not decompose easily they eventually produce significant quantities of biomass. Since mango leaves are commonly available they have not yet become commercialized.

Mango fruit is a great source of income for all households especially if you have access to those growing 'wild'.

Goats love the leaves. This could be hazardous to the tree during the early growing stages, but once the tree is established the occasional nibble from the goat does it no harm.

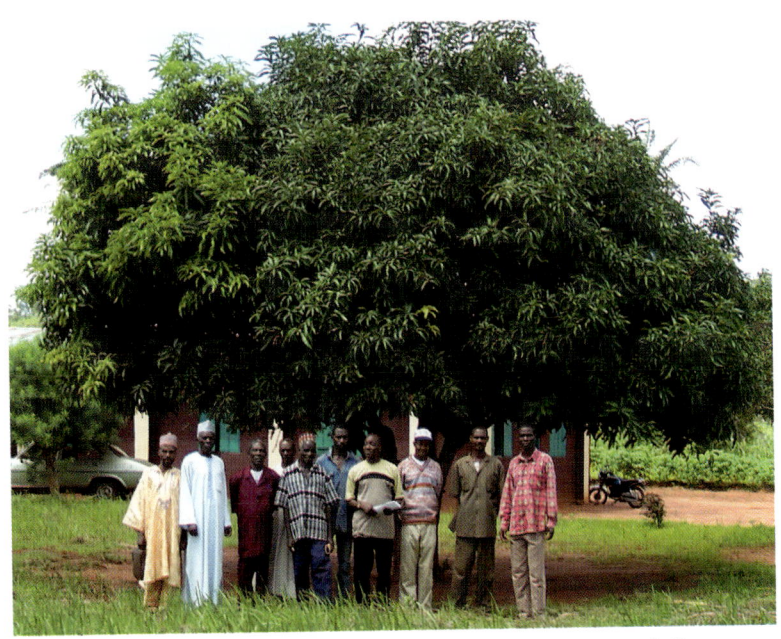

What better shade than that of a mango especially during the noon day sun. It is a forest tree that lends much enchantment and coolness to its surroundings.

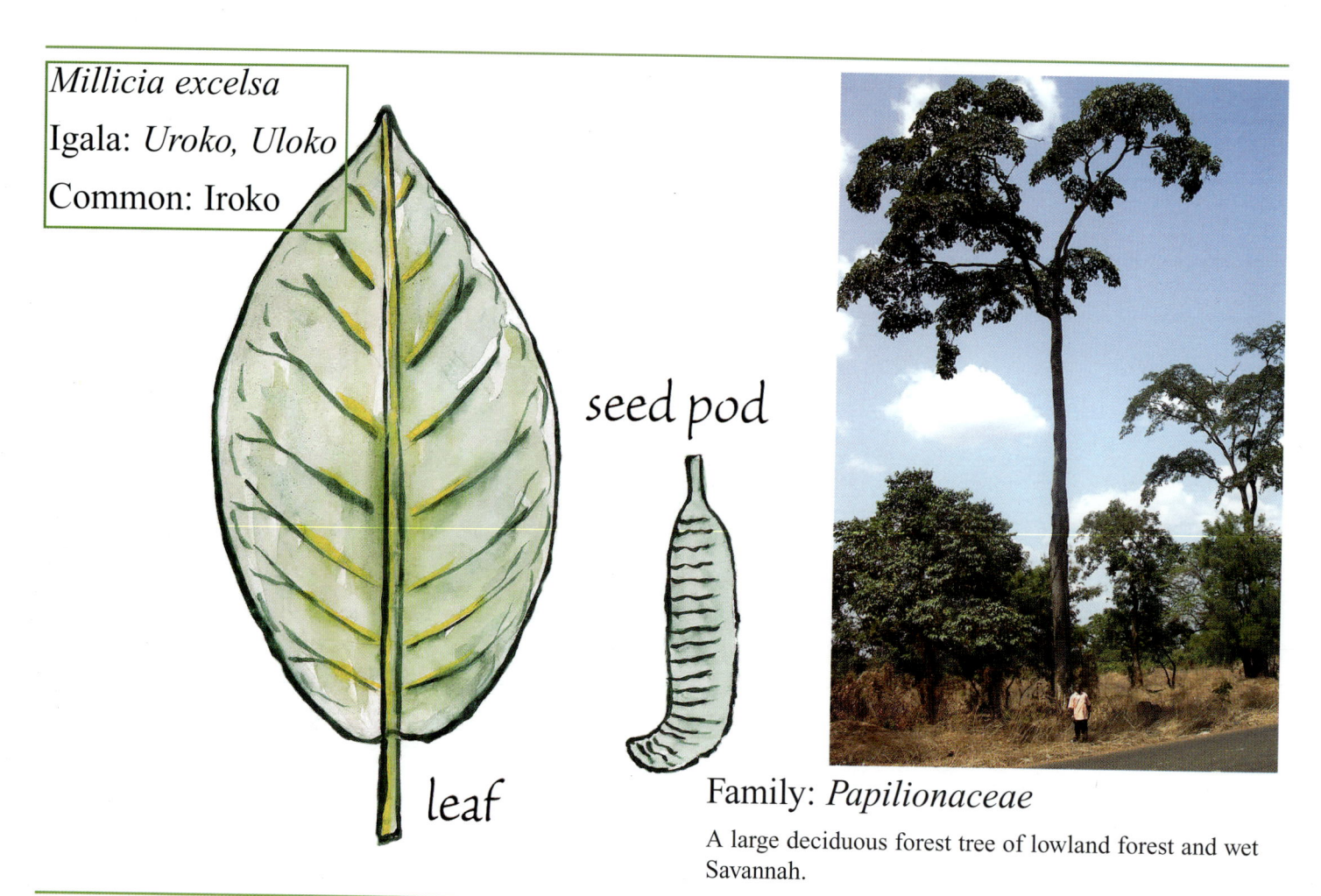

Millicia excelsa
Igala: *Uroko, Uloko*
Common: Iroko

leaf

seed pod

Family: *Papilionaceae*

A large deciduous forest tree of lowland forest and wet Savannah.

•Food

Iroko has no use as a food.

•Cultural

Iroko is a hard wood and greatly prized throughout the region and the continent as a whole. Little wonder it is referred to as the King of Hardwood Trees.

Traditional believers worship it as their idol, and also worship the image as their god.

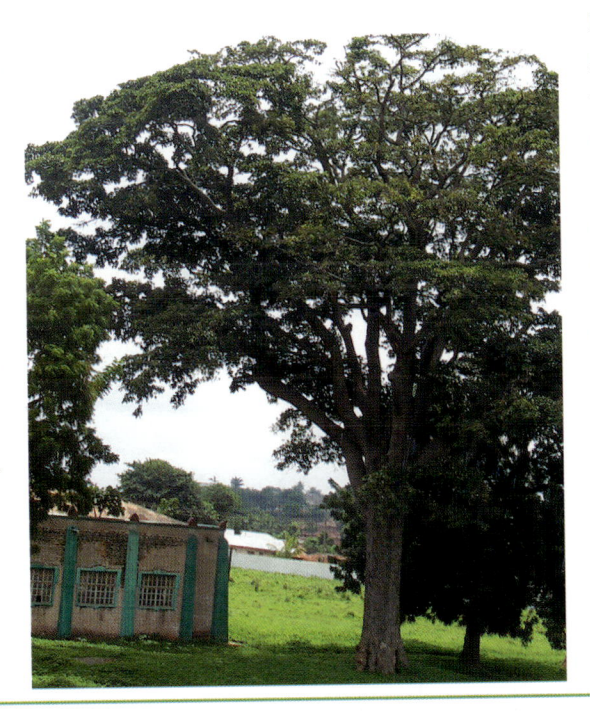

Elders use it as a place of sacrifice to their gods. No one dares go near it at night.

People burn the wood along farm headlands believing this clears away evil spirits. The bark, when put in a fire, drives away evil spirits and it is also used in guarding the farm.

Traditional images for ceremonial use are carved from the wood.

There is a local belief that witches and wizards will not approach this tree, therefore people endeavour to have it in their compounds. This is now more difficult as the tree becomes scarcer due to its popularity as a cash crop.

A tree climber will never climb this tree. No other tree can ever overshadow it.

Iroko tree in the Attah of Igala's palace compound, Idah

Oli bibi kegbe makobojinia.
No matter how strong is a particular tree, it cannot overshadow *ukolo*.

•Medicinal

The root is used as an antidote for snakebite if mixed with *abo* and *aloko* roots and snake's head. All are ground to a paste and applied externally to the affected area.

The same root and bark if pounded to a paste cures oedema. It is also applied externally.

If iroko and *Ogęlę* roots are mixed and boiled, the medicine can cure convulsions. The patient bathes in the liquid and there is no oral treatment.

The leaves when boiled cure dysentery. Dosage: 1 glass 3 times a day for 7 days.

The leaves of iroko and *Ogęlę* are boiled and liquid taken for stomach pain. Dosage: 1 glass 3 times a day for 7 days.

To cure malaria and skin diseases, leaves and bark of iroko are boiled and used twice daily for bathing only.

Chairs made of iroko wood

•Other uses

Iroko, noted worldwide as the premier hardwood for furniture, is now highly endangered in this region. Because the wood is exported, very few local people can afford to buy it. However, it is much coveted for traditional and local buildings.

Varnishing picks up the natural grain in the wood which has resistance to woodworm.

Iroko is acknowledged as a superb firewood but this luxury is rarely available.

Nowadays only wood rejected by sawmills is used to make handles and farm implements.

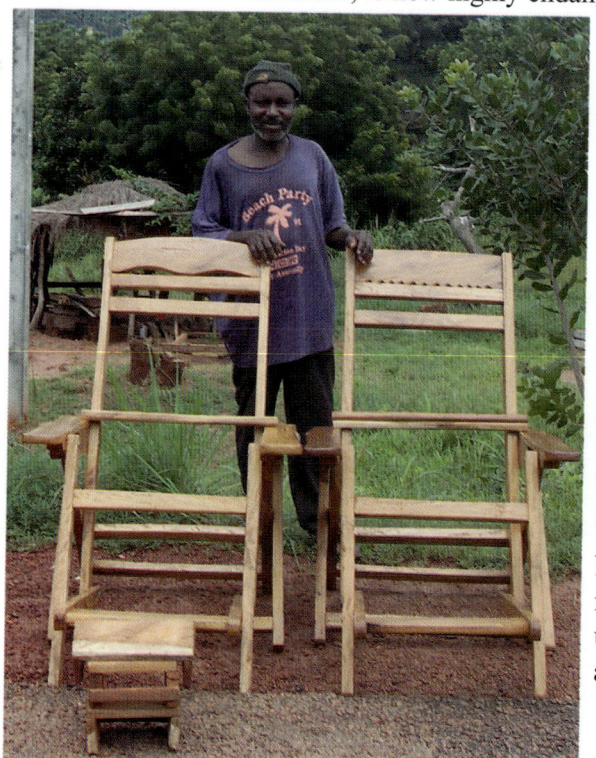

Also suitable for trucks and backs of lorries.

As a source of good biomass, *Iroko* enhances soil fertility.

Because it grows so tall it is not always effective for shade. However, its numerous branches lend solace to passers by before it grows too tall.

Goats eat the leaves that fall from its lofty heights.

Presently not too much money is generated from it because it has become so scarce. Unfortunately little replanting is being done.

Iroko's appearance can best be described as regal.

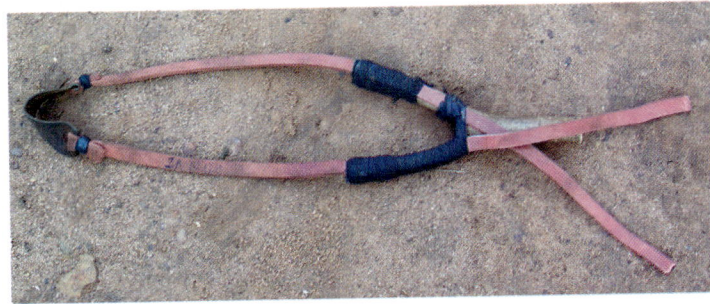

Child's catapult

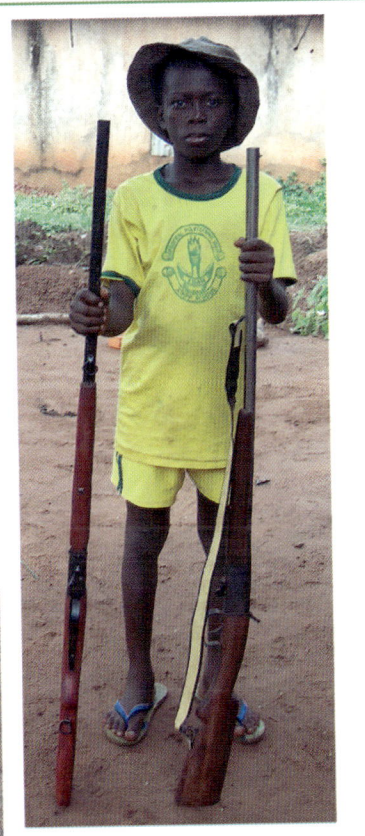

Dane guns made in part from *iroko* wood

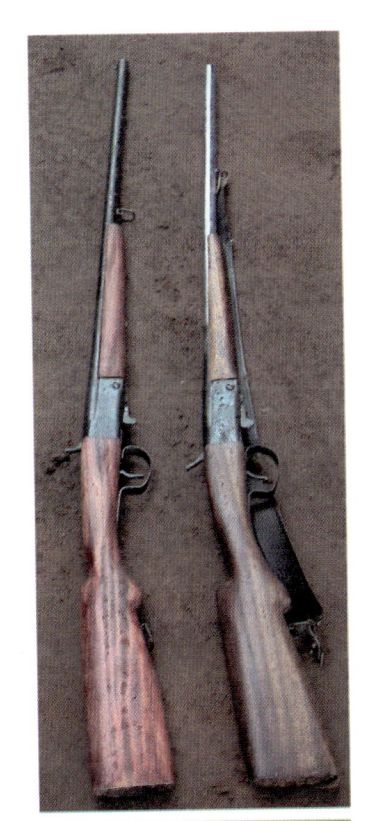

Mitragyna inermis

Igala: *Ọtọchi*

Common: Iroko

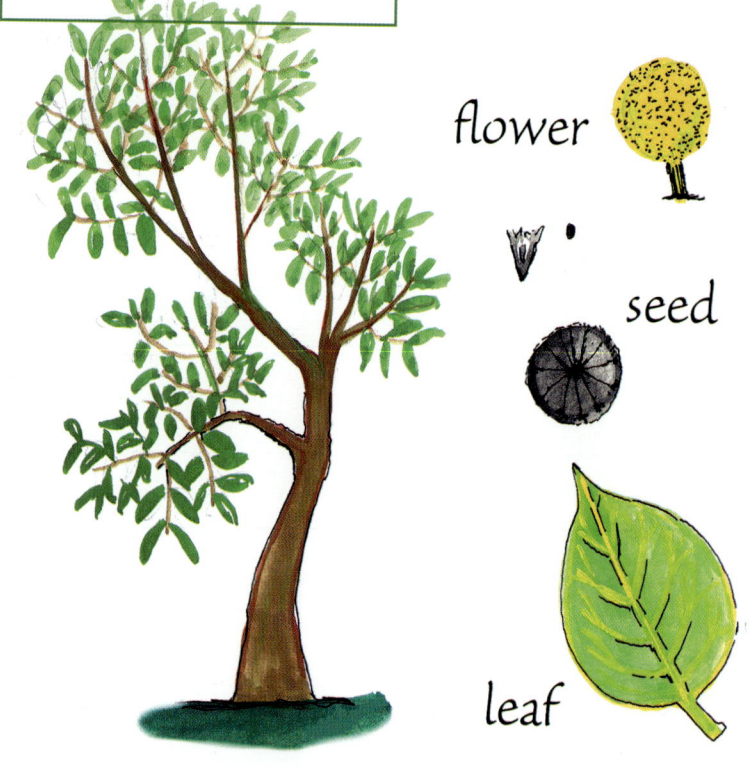

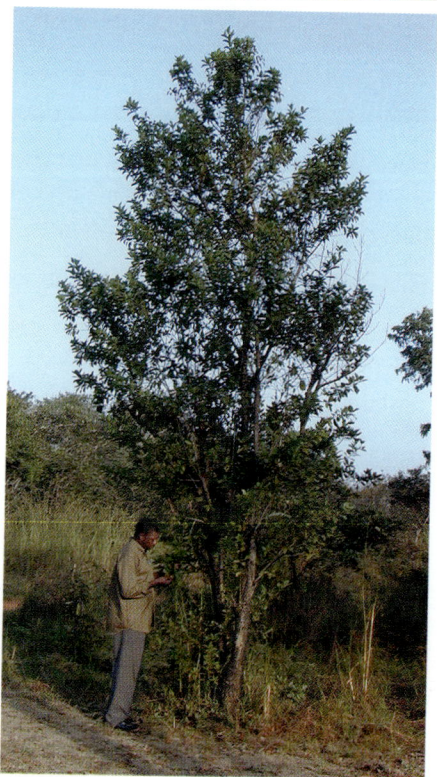

flower

seed

leaf

Family: *Rubiaceae*

A shrub or low branching tree growing up to 20 to 40 ft high. Has a scaly bark and yellow-white flower heads. Usually found on clay soils in savannah areas.

- **Food**

Not used for food.

- **Cultural**

Its shade serves as a worshipping ground.

- **Medicinal**

Otochi cures dysentery. Its leaves and bark are boiled with leaves and bark of rosewood, and the medicine taken 3 times daily for 7 days. The same medicine cures all fevers and back ache.

Otochi root provides an antidote for certain poisons.

- **Other uses**

Grown mainly in the riverine areas, as fuel it is not as long lasting as *ugba* and *Orachi*. However, women prefer it to other types of firewood because it lights easily with a large flame, similar to gmelina.

This housewife selects and arranges firewood

Otochi wood is used for making traditional seats, paddles, idols, pestles, door frames, handles for all agricultural tools, as well as frames and roofing sticks for local houses, *atakpas* and kitchens. All sell well in local markets.

It also rates highly as a fertilizer tree because it enriches the soil.

Though rarely found in compounds, farmers like it on their farms as beneath its shade they often take a rest and store their farm produce before transporting it to their compounds. Farmers buy branches as staking sticks.

Otochi bark, roots and leaves are purchased for their medicinal properties. Goats like the leaves and bark but this can cause damage to the tree. An abundance of this tree is admirable guaranteeing a therapeutic ambience.

Morinda lucida

Igala: *Ọgẹlẹ*

Common: Bonko fruit

leaf

fruit

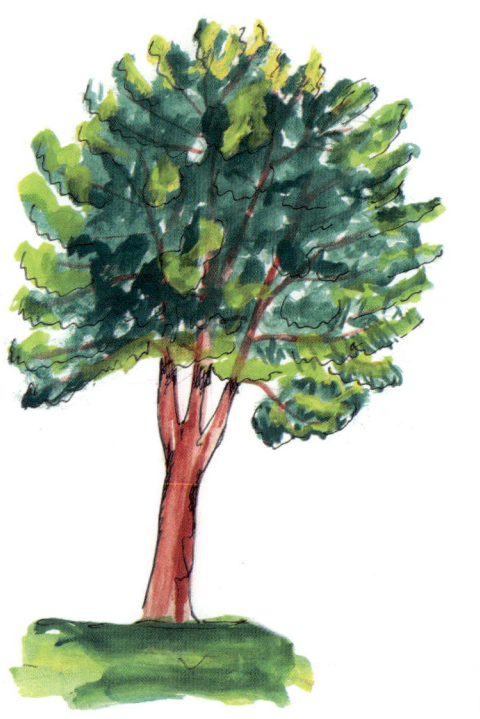

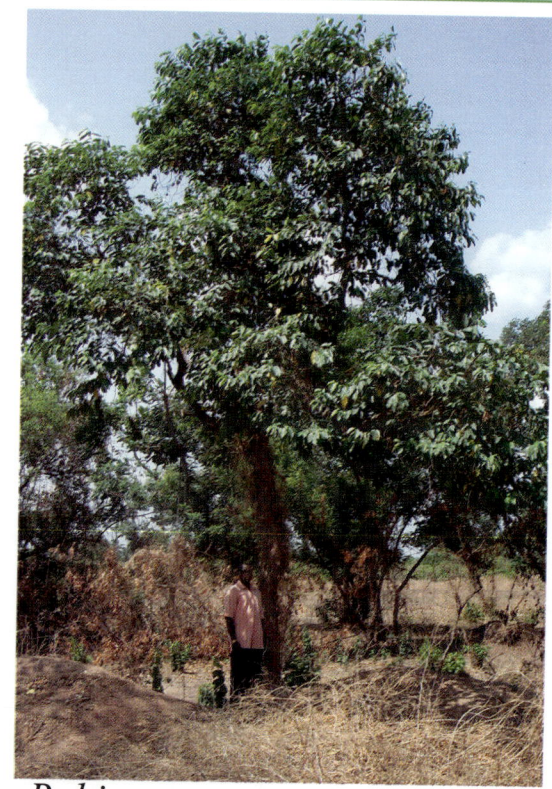

Family: *Rubiaceae*

A medium-sized tree with scaly grey bark and short branches. Flowers are white and occur in small heads. Fruits are green with a white interior.

•Food

No value as food.

•Cultural

Beneath its shade a worshipping-ground is found, as this picture depicts.

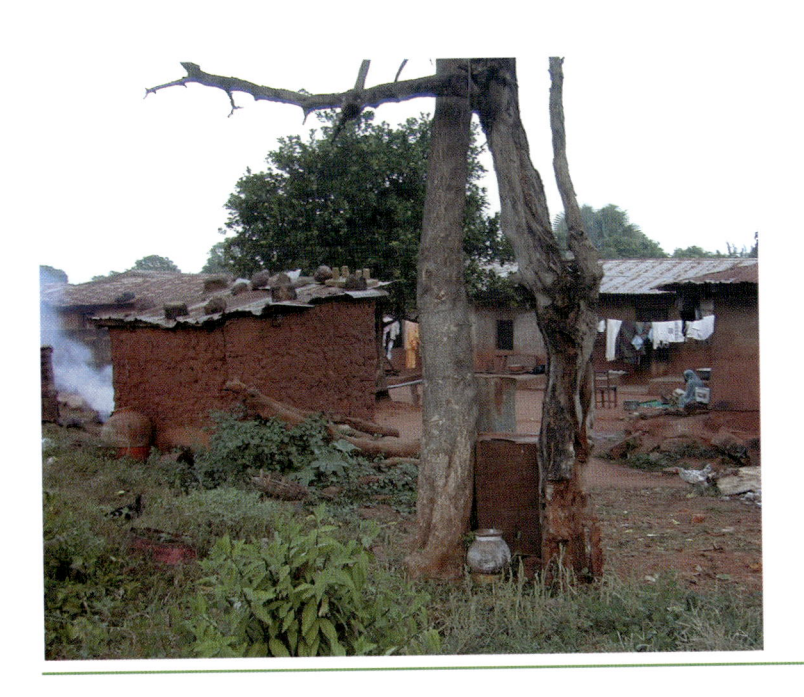

If the owner places these leaves on top of properties it protects against thieves. The dire consequences for an offender is convulsions in his/her children.

•Medicinal

As a cure for stomach ache in infants the leaves are rubbed and the little liquid extracted given to the infant. Because of its bitterness, dosage is one drop 3 times daily for 7 or 14 days. For adults with stomach ache the leaves are soaked in water and 1 glass taken cold 3 times daily.

For convulsions, *Ogẹlẹ* and *Ugba* leaves are combined and boiled. The liquid can be used for bathing. This is only taken once, warmed before being swallowed. It also cures malaria, coughs and sore throats. Dosage: 1 glass 3 times daily for 7 days.

To cure ear problems, bark and leaves are boiled and a drop put in the ear 3 times daily for 7 days.

•Other uses

Ọgẹlẹ is such an excellent firewood that women travel any distance to find it. A fire made from Ọgẹlẹ wood lasts a couple days. Now endangered, the Ọgẹlẹ tree is not being replanted at a desirable rate.

Although considered suitable for domestic and office furniture, it is difficult to get a trunk that gives the right size planks. However, when planks are available they require little paint or varnish. Ọgẹlẹ also has resistance to woodworm.

Its lighter branches are good as staking sticks that last for some years. This saves labour, a scarce commodity in this region.

Traditional seats and handles for all agricultural tools including spades, are amongst the many uses of Ọgẹlẹ wood.

Its fork stick and trunk are used for local houses, *atakpas* and kitchens. The wood is particularly good for roofing.

Carvers use it to craft idols and other ceremonial images.

Ọgẹlẹ has a reputation for enhancing soil fertility with its lavish biomass. As it does not grow too tall, it has good shade and looks attractive when in flower.

Goats enjoy the tree but can easily damage it; owners therefore protect it from animals.

Ọgẹlẹ planks and roofing materials are always in high demand and fetch good revenue. Much of the wood is exported. Men only sell the wood, and women its leaves for medicinal use.

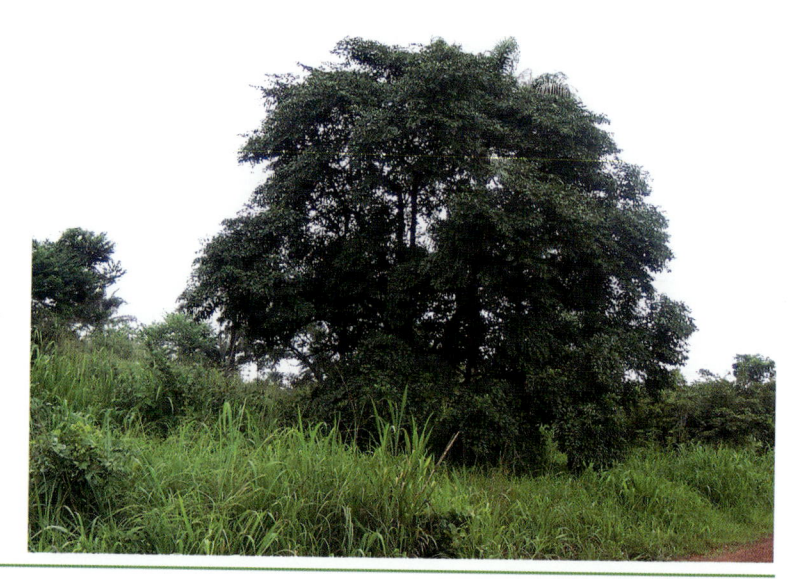

Newbouldia laevis

Igala: *Ogichi*

Common: African Border Tree

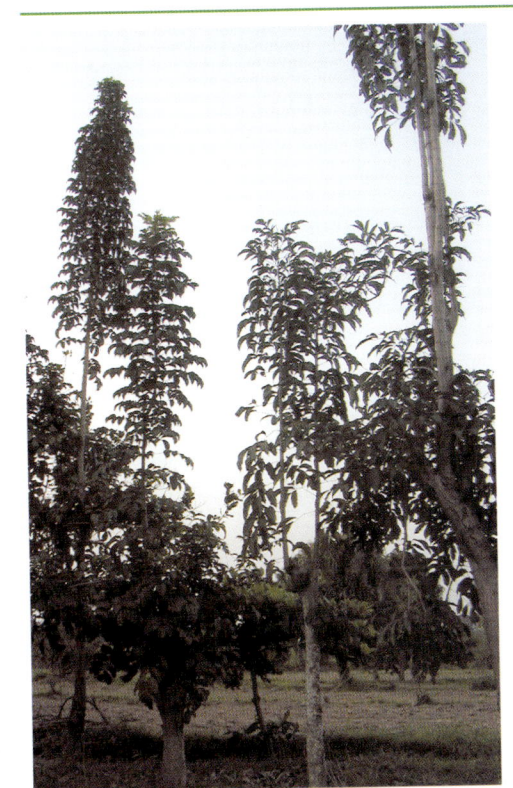

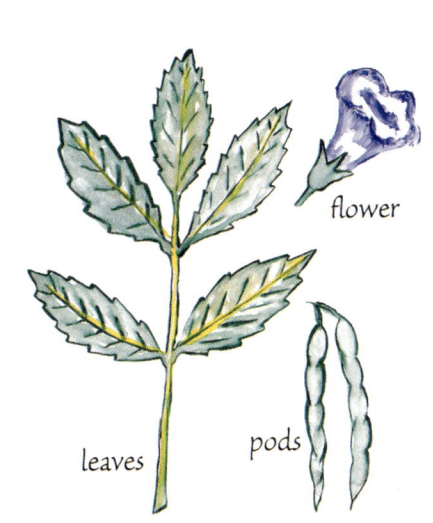

Family: *Bignoniaceae*

Medium sized tree usually slender in form and growing up to 40 ft tall. Flowers are red-purple or pink and white in colour. Commonly found in villages and towns as boundary demarcation.

leaves flower pods

113

•Food

The liquid content of its flower eaten by children as a snack often relieves their hunger pangs.

•Cultural

This tree is generally associated with marking boundaries and constructing sturdy fences. In turn its rich biomass fertilizes the plots it demarcates.

The *ogichi* indicates the location of graves.

Often used as a staking stick for yam it lasts for many years – an important factor in a region where labour is at a premium.

Like the neem tree, Moslems spread the leaves of the *ogichi* tree on top of a frame to protect a body being laid to rest. This ensures the earth does not fall directly onto the body.

Ogichi is sometimes used to construct local shrines.

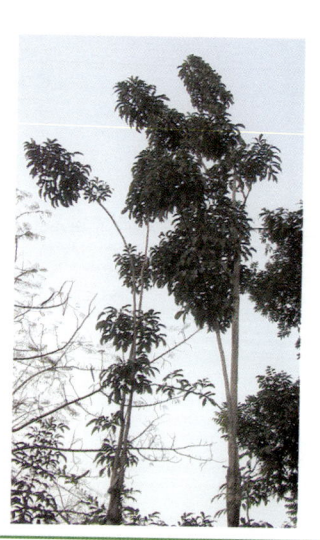

•Medicinal

To relieve labour pains, *ogichi* leaves are squeezed in cold water; the liquid is then given to women in labour. There is no specific dosage.

A sick baby can be helped when *ogichi* leaves are boiled with guava and lime leaves. The infant is given a drop of this medicine 3 times daily. The remainder is used for the baby's bath.

Ogichi is a known cure for all categories of fever, especially malaria, typhoid, jaundice (yellow fever) and all other related illnesses. Leaves are boiled and 1 glass taken 3 times daily for 7 days, and the remainder used for bathing.

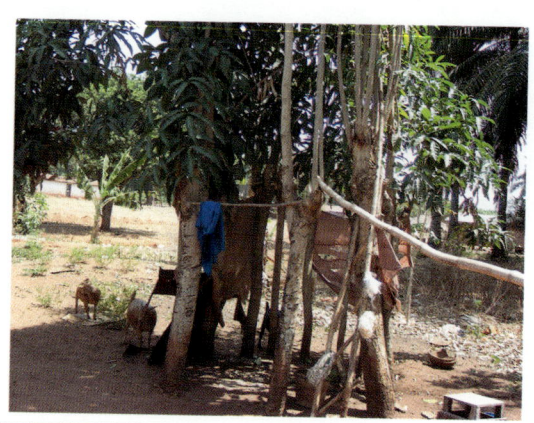

Coughs and sore throats are cured by chewing the stem.

•Other uses

Ogichi is regularly used for firewood and still plentiful.

Its fork stick is used for constructing granaries, *atakpas* and kitchens, and its live sticks for building yam barns.

Handles for cutlasses and local knives are produced from it.

Ogichi leaves decompose easily and so improve the condition of the soil. This is an extra bonus when it is used as a boundary demarcation as the organic matter can be transferred easily to the plots it marks.

Ogichi provides one of the most useful forms of low shade although it can grow up to three metres.

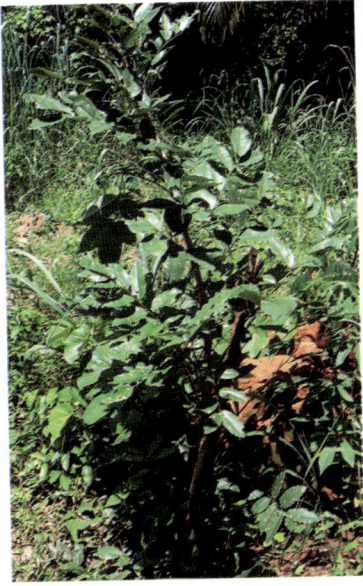

Ogichi easily propagates by cutting and passed from neighbour to neighbour free of charge.

Its attractive flowers add to a garden looking neat and compact with *ogichi* fencing a good bio experience.

Goats are given *ogichi* leaves to eat after kidding to reduce complications.

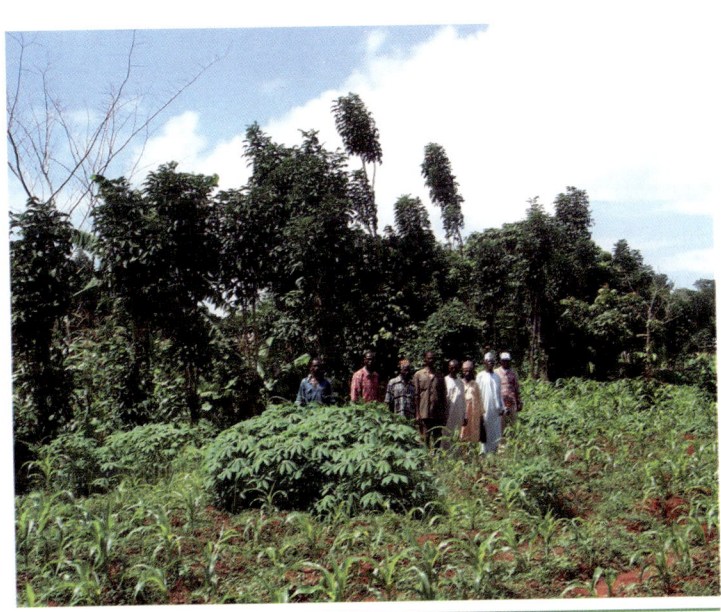

Parkia biglobsa

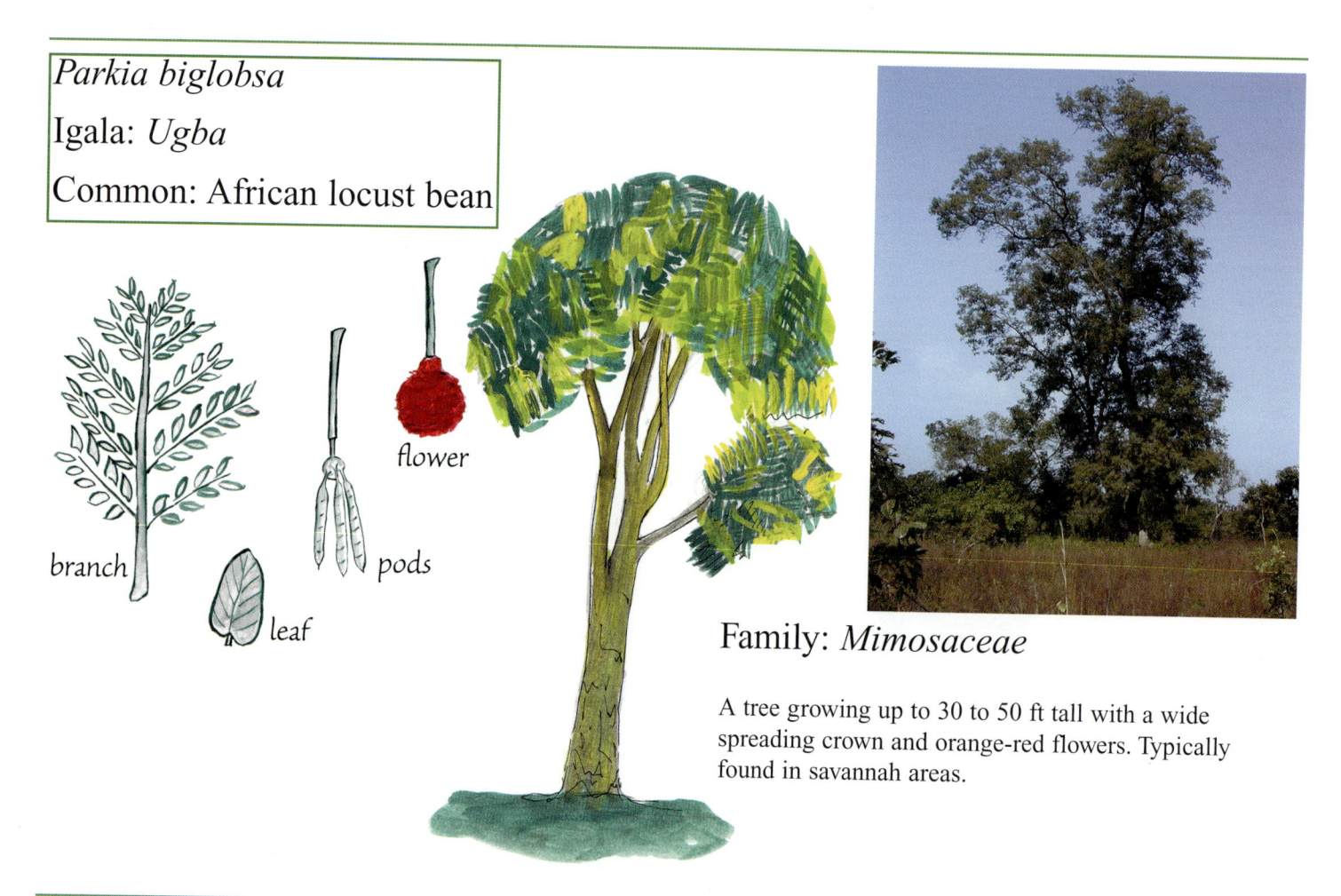

Igala: *Ugba*

Common: African locust bean

branch

leaf

flower

pods

Family: *Mimosaceae*

A tree growing up to 30 to 50 ft tall with a wide spreading crown and orange-red flowers. Typically found in savannah areas.

•Food

Traditionally it is the main soup ingredient, as soup has no taste without it. Ashes from its dried wood are also used for local soup.

•Cultural

Ugba acts as a thief deterrent if you place the dry wood on top of your belongings. Anyone stealing property thus protected swells all over and there is no cure. No cases have been recorded recently.

A former use, but now out of date, was to apply it to make a person smell badly – believed to cause bad luck!

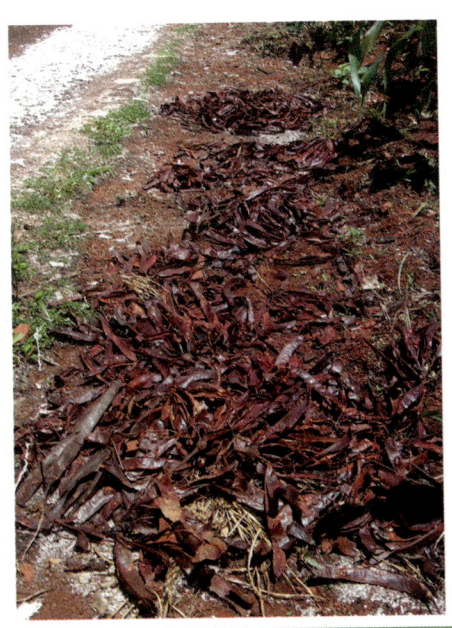

•Medicinal

The bark can be chewed to get rid of bad breath.

To ease labour pains, the leaves and bark are boiled. Dosage: 1 glass 3 times daily for 3 months before the expected time of delivery.

To relieve stomach ache, fold the leaves and boil with the bark. Dosage: 1 glass 3 times daily for 7 days.

To cure convulsions, leaves are boiled with *ebe* (a grass). Dosage: 1 glass 3 times daily and some of the medicine is used for bathing the patient. Another combination for curing convulsion is to boil *ugba* and *Ogẹlẹ* leaves and then divide the liquid. Part is drunk at the dose rate of 1 glass twice daily over 7 days; the remainder is used for bathing.

Soap made from locust bean ashes is used for treatment of skin disease.

In picture: *Ugba pods* left to dry on the side of a tarred road – a convenient, if dangerous, spot for such a purpose! The white material on the road is cassava flour – also placed there for drying.

•Other uses

Ugba is now endangered in some areas, despite being one of the trees that is most easily self-propagated.

Housewives like its firewood, but rarely use it because of its other benefits.

Carvers enjoy it in crafting images for traditional worship and local festivals.

Because it has a very good fork stick, it has become a great favourite for granaries, *atakpas*, frames for local buildings, handles for hoes, cutlasses, axes; mortars and pestles are carved from it.

The richness of the soil in areas with *ugba* is testimony to the effectiveness of leguminous trees. Locust trees certainly merit its local name, Fertilizer Tree.

It grows tall slowly, and on reaching its maximum height provides little shade.

As it does not absorb or retain moisture it is a premier firewood and valued for the revenue it generates.

The seed value in the market is high because it is the main ingredient used in the production of *Magi* (stock cubes), a cash crop exported to the north of Nigeria.

The leaves and bark have a high market value because of their medicinal use, as has the soap made from it.

Ọlabimẹ dabọ olabi ugba – Your bad luck is such that people are scared away from you.

Ukpekpele manyugba, ugbatakpa uludọmọ – The odour of the calabash used to process Ugba into magi remains in people long after it is consumed

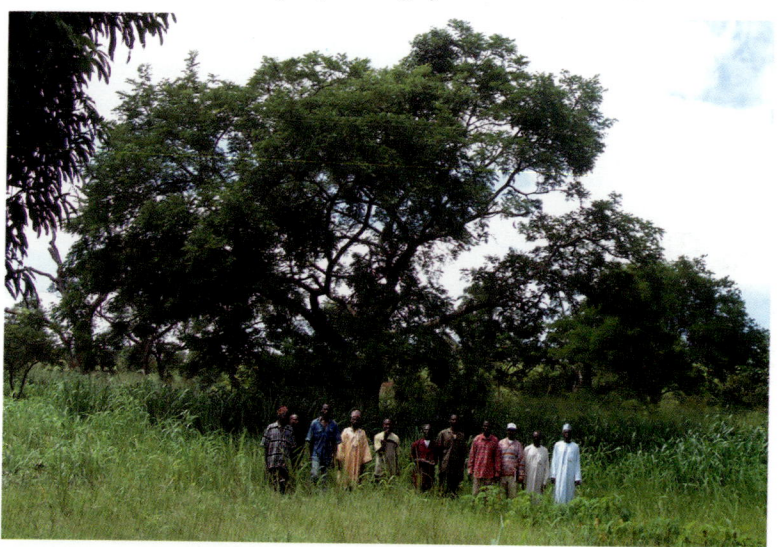

Persea americana

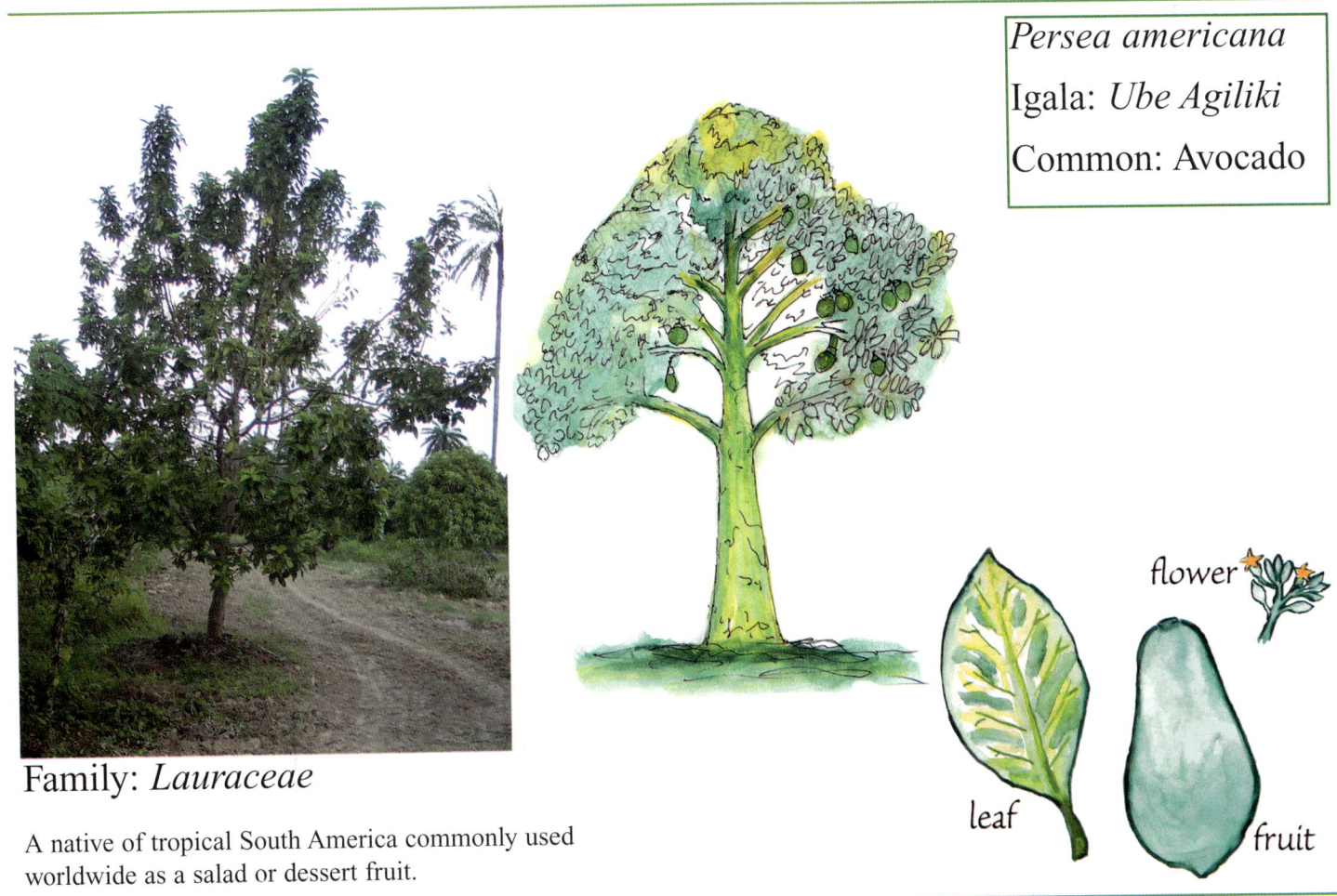

Igala: *Ube Agiliki*

Common: Avocado

Family: *Lauraceae*

A native of tropical South America commonly used worldwide as a salad or dessert fruit.

leaf flower fruit

119

- **Food**

Its fruit is edible and rich in Vitamin E.

- **Cultural**

Its leaves are used to scare thieves. If folded and placed on property no one dares touch it.

The avocado has only recently made its debut in this region. This is a sign of hope and life as it enriches and extends the region's natural resource base.

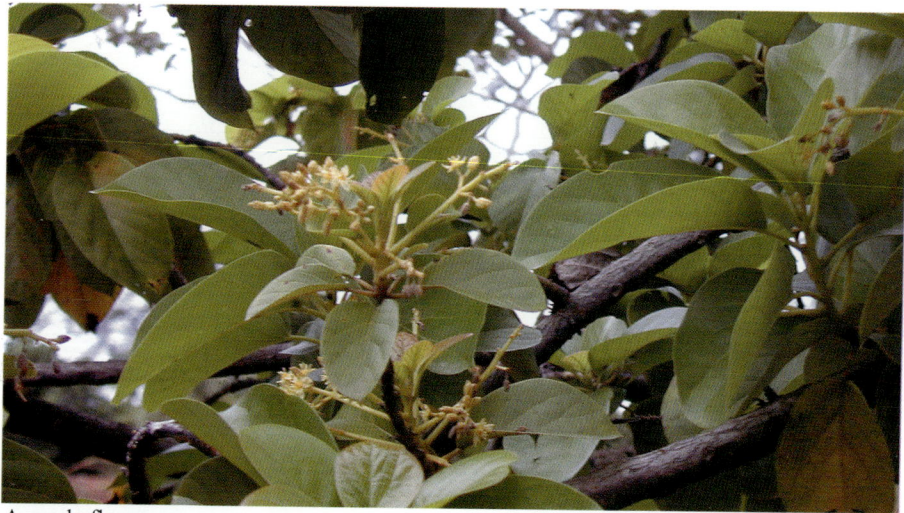

Avocado flowers

- **Medicinal**

Avocado has no known medicinal properties.

- **Other uses**

Even though it is a newcomer in the region, no one likes to cut it for firewood because of the fruit's value

After many years the tree develops a substantial trunk which, when sawn into planks, is suitable for all furniture. Although the avocado tree produces fork sticks no one uses it for this purpose, except when the tree dies as result of drought.

The tree needs good soil conditions.

Avocado bears leaves all year round but it takes years to grow tall, a fact valued for fruit picking.

The fruit, now valuable, is being developed as a cash crop.

Those who raise it protect it from goats.

Phyllanthus discoides
Igala: *Ode*
Common: Makarara

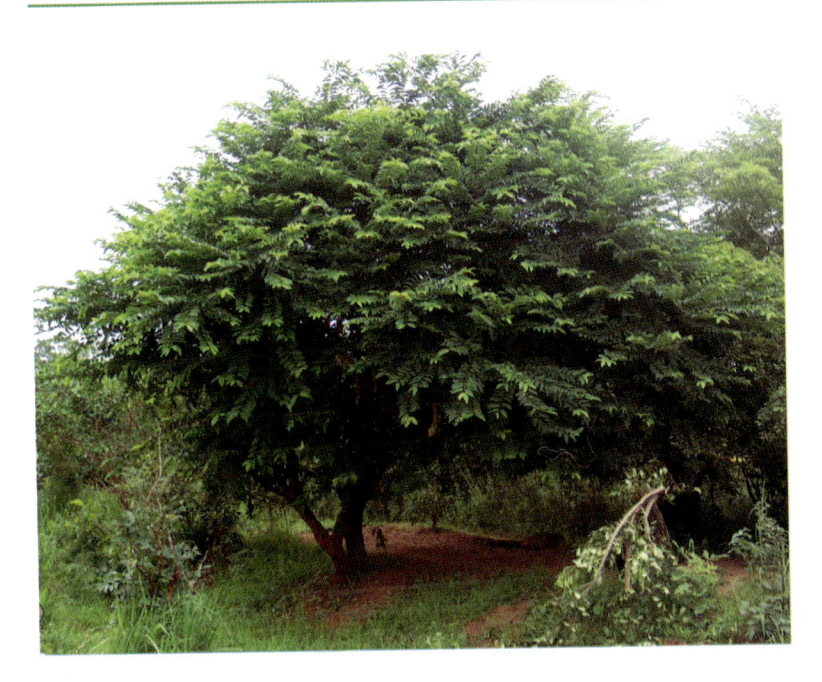

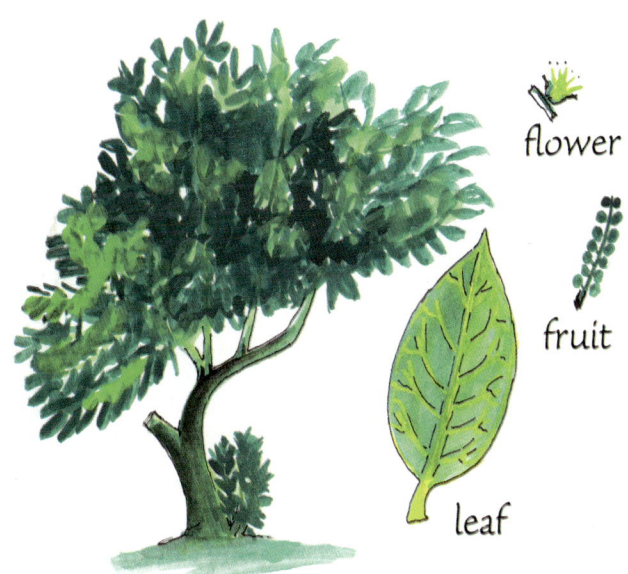

Family: *Euphorbiaceae*

Large deciduous shrub or tree, growing up to 100 ft tall. Found in moister parts of savannah or drier parts of forest. Flowers are yellow-green.

flower

fruit

leaf

•Food

Nothing edible from *Ode*.

•Cultural

Not used for cultural purposes.

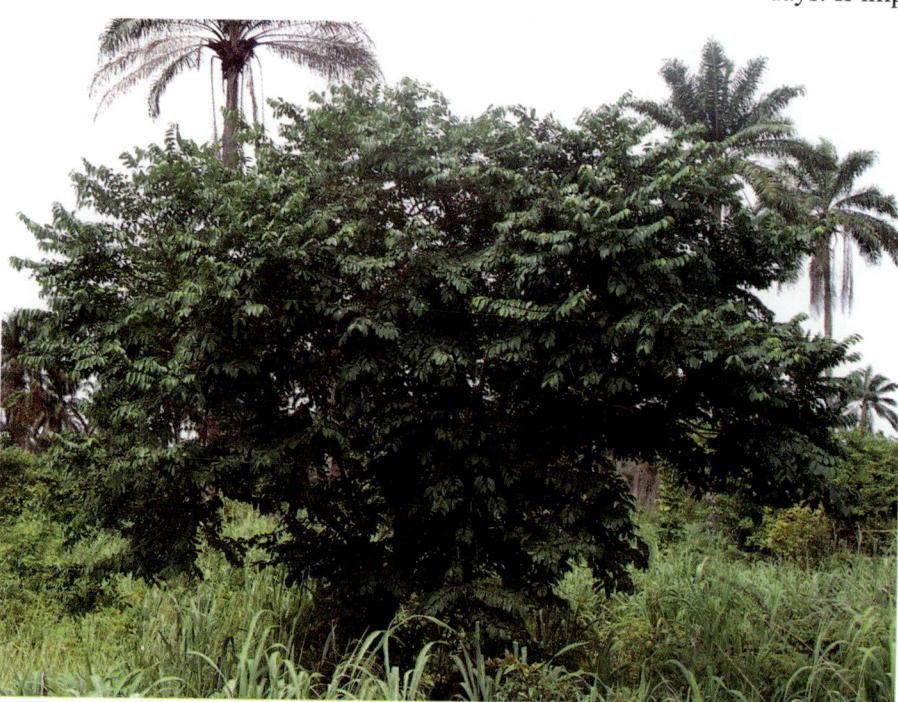

•Medicinal

To cure waist and rheumatic pains, pound the barks of *ode, ejiji, andayigẹlẹ* and *ayinyili* seed to a paste. Mould into small round portions and sun-dry. Grind and then mix with water. Dosage: 1 glass 3 times a day for 7 days. If impossible to grind, the portions can be dissolved in local gin, and 1 small glass taken 3 times daily for 7 days.

To cure backache, combine *ode* and *Ọgẹlẹ* barks and *alu* (fruit) and grind to a paste with water. Take twice daily for 7 days.

To help give strength to women in early pregnancy, grind *ode* and *ogbogbo* barks to a paste and dilute with cold water. Dosage: 1 glass taken twice daily. The rest of the paste is applied to the body at bedtime.

•Other uses

Not used for other purposes.

Podococcus barteri
Igala: *Odo*
Common: Fan palm

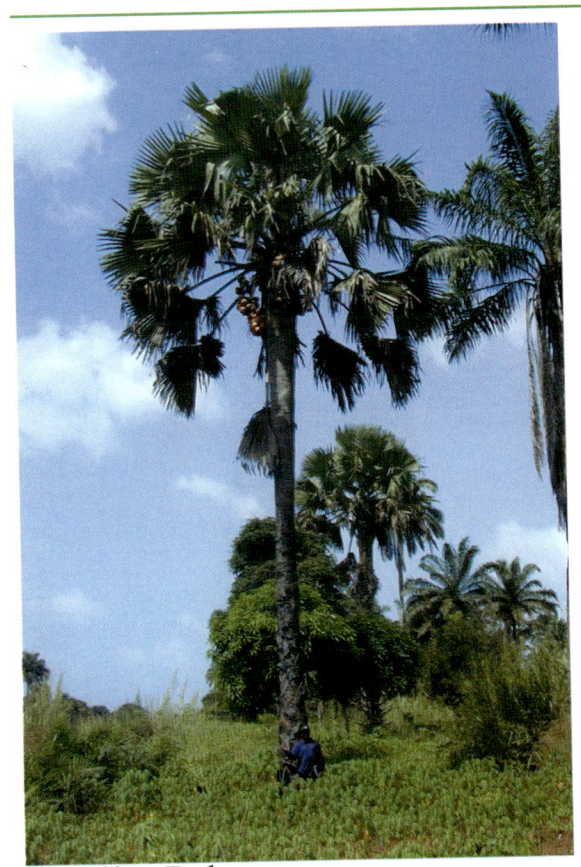

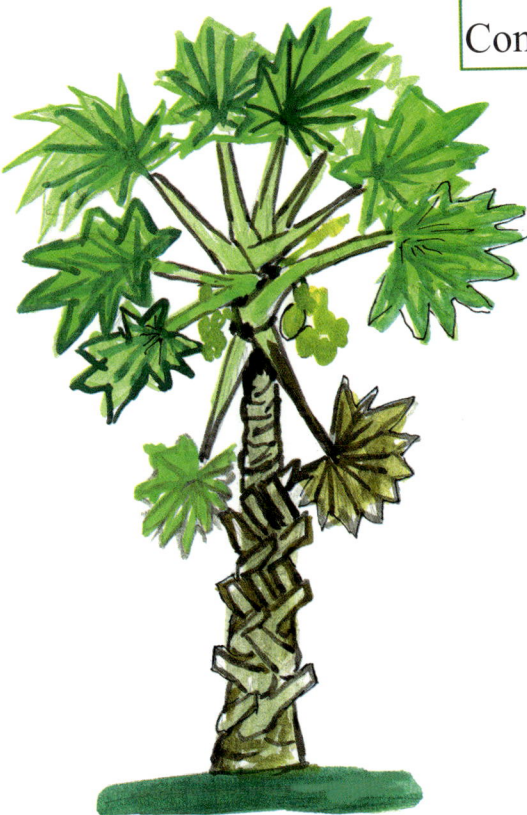

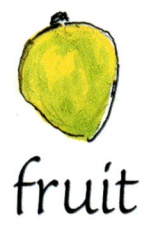

Family: Palmae
A slender and elegant palm with orange-red fruits.

fruit

123

•Food

The fruit and nut are edible and sold in the markets at a high price. Women trade in these commodities.

If the fruit is buried in the soil it produces a tuber which can be eaten like yam, a luxury and difficult to find. Its liquid part is used to prepare pap.

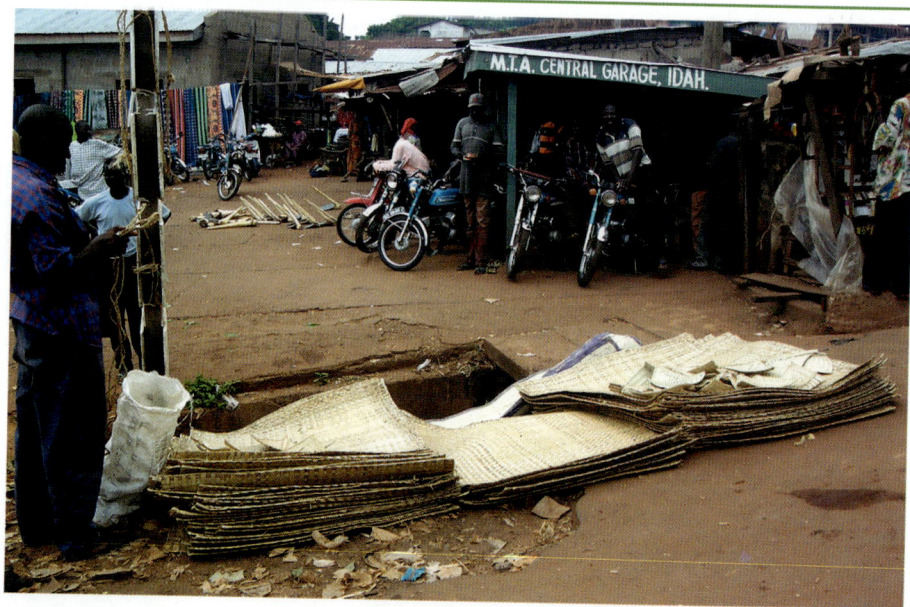

•Cultural

Odo is used in making mats for traditional burials. This mat also assumes importance during traditional marriages when the wife to be and a relative of the husband to be sit on it while cola is being presented to the in-laws. It is then left in front of the ancestral idols to intercede for the couple.

This type of mat is hung over doorposts of the ancestral worship houses.

Odo mats for sale in Idah market

•Medicinal

It produces a type of wine which contains yeast often used for treating eyes; part is rubbed onto the eyes and part drunk.

It is also administered to children with measles, rubbed onto the body to bring out the rash, giving relief to the patient.

Just like palm wine, it acts as an antidote to all types of poison; part is taken orally with the remainder rubbed on the body.

Barren women use the root to become pregnant. The root is boiled with spear grass and 1 glass taken 3 times daily for as long as necessary.

Some men with poor ejaculation use the fruit which has to fall naturally to the ground; it produces a tuber which the patient eats raw.

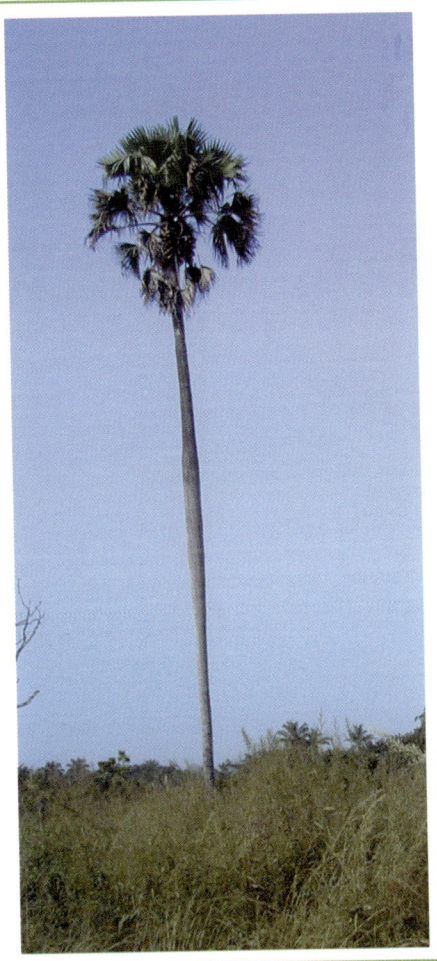

•Other uses

The branches and trunk are used for firewood.

Not used to make furniture, but local drums are made from it.

The trunk is acknowledged as among the best roofing wood in the region. Before the chain saw was introduced it was used for all roofing and frames for local dwelling houses. The leaves provided the thatch.

The leaves are suitable for erosion control and the manufacture of local fans and mats.

When the tree dies its residue is extremely valuable as a soil nutrient which enhances fruit production.

A very lucrative wood; its wine is also expensive.

It is extremely majestic especially when laden with a crop of its red fruit. Its great height makes it ineffective as shade (see pic).

Children use the hairy part of the seed to practice plaiting hair.

Prosopis africana

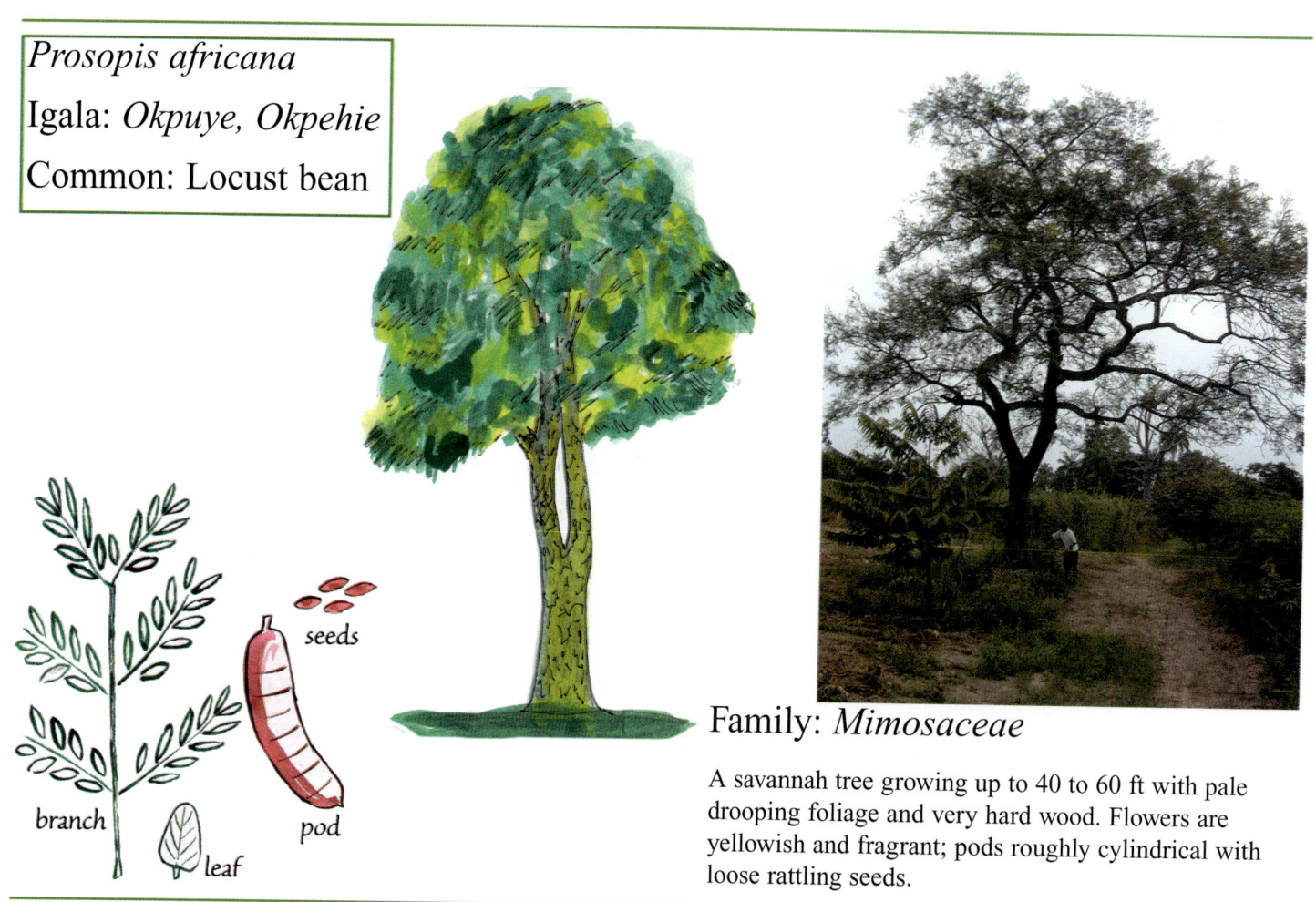

Igala: *Okpuye, Okpehie*

Common: Locust bean

branch, leaf, pod, seeds

Family: *Mimosaceae*

A savannah tree growing up to 40 to 60 ft with pale drooping foliage and very hard wood. Flowers are yellowish and fragrant; pods roughly cylindrical with loose rattling seeds.

•Food

The seed is used as local *Magi* (stock cube).

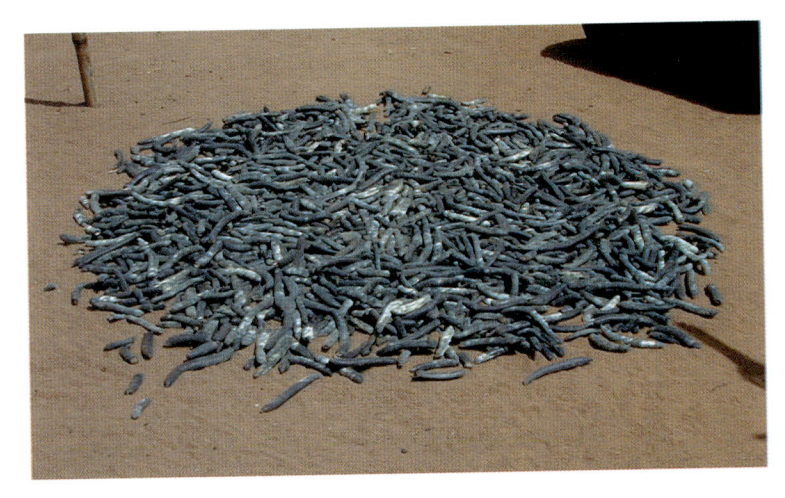

•Medicinal

The leaves boiled with *Ogẹlẹ* (*Morinda lucida*) are used to treat convulsions, fever and headache.

•Cultural

The firewood is used in identifying wrongdoers in society, especially those who refuse to admit their offense.

To perform the ceremony its wood is set alight. A spade placed in the centre of the fire is heated to 100°c. When red-hot a ceremony is performed in a pot, and a liquid from this ritual given to the suspect to drink. The person is next expected to wash his/her face and mouth with this potion, and afterwards instructed to pick the red-hot spade from the fire with his/her teeth and then dip it in the ceremonial liquid in the pot. If the suspect is guilty the flame will rise, but if innocent the flame will reduce drastically allowing the suspect to pick the spade with his/her teeth.

There were witnesses to such a ceremony in 1982 when a contribution to a local rotational saving fund was stolen. The suspect was identified and confessed to his theft. The stolen money was returned. He also had to pay a community fine as well as providing a ram and drinks for entertainment.

•Other uses

The wood, strong and long lasting, is popular as firewood. The pods when used also quickly kindle the fire.

Blacksmiths use the wood as charcoal in their forges.

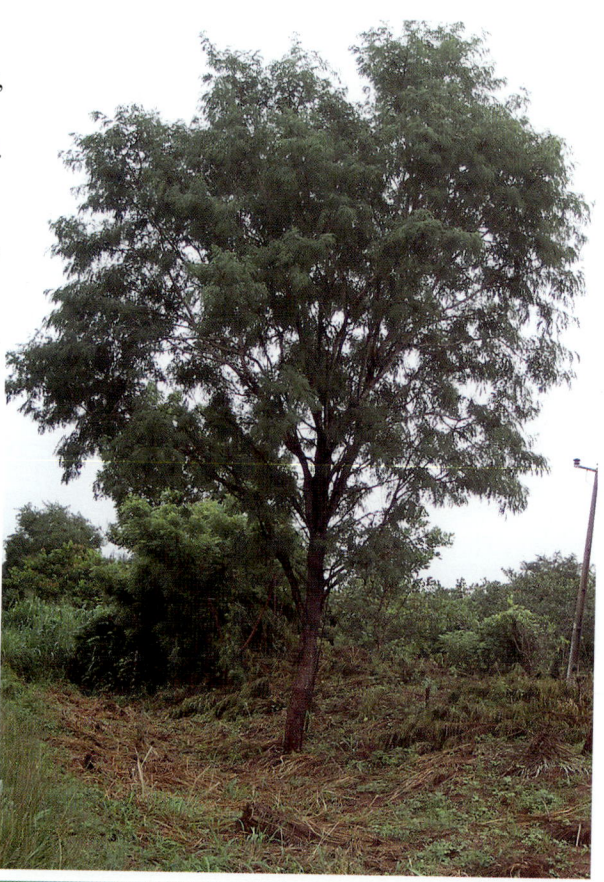

Artists carve images from it. Mortars and pestles, handles for farm implements, frames for local houses, granaries, kitchens, pillars for verandahs and chewing sticks are made from its wood. The dry wood is preferred to the newly sawn because of its resistance to wood worm.

The locust bean tree provides excellent shade. Anything planted close by thrives and it is valued for its nitrogenous properties (it fixes nitrogen from the atmosphere). This earns it the name Fertilizer Tree. Its decaying leaves further improves fertility. It is one of the farmer's best friends.

Goats eat the beans and the red flowers that fall to the ground. Given the opportunity, they also eat the leaves but this can damage young trees.

Growing more gracious as it ages, towering into the sky, it provides a background for the other vegetation it helps nourish.

It is also a good money spinner because the bean processed into a local form of *Magi* (stock cube) has great export value.

Psidium guajava

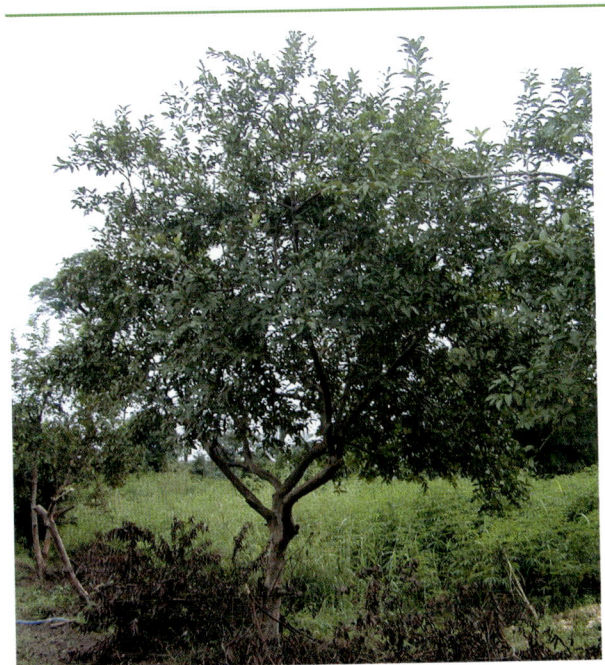

Igala: *Igwoba*

Common: Guava

Family: *Myrtaceae*

Shrub or small tree, native of American tropics, growing up to 30 feet tall, with scaly, green-brown bark, large leaves and white flowers. Fruit is ovoid to pear-shaped, 1 to 4 inches long, with yellow or dark pink flesh.

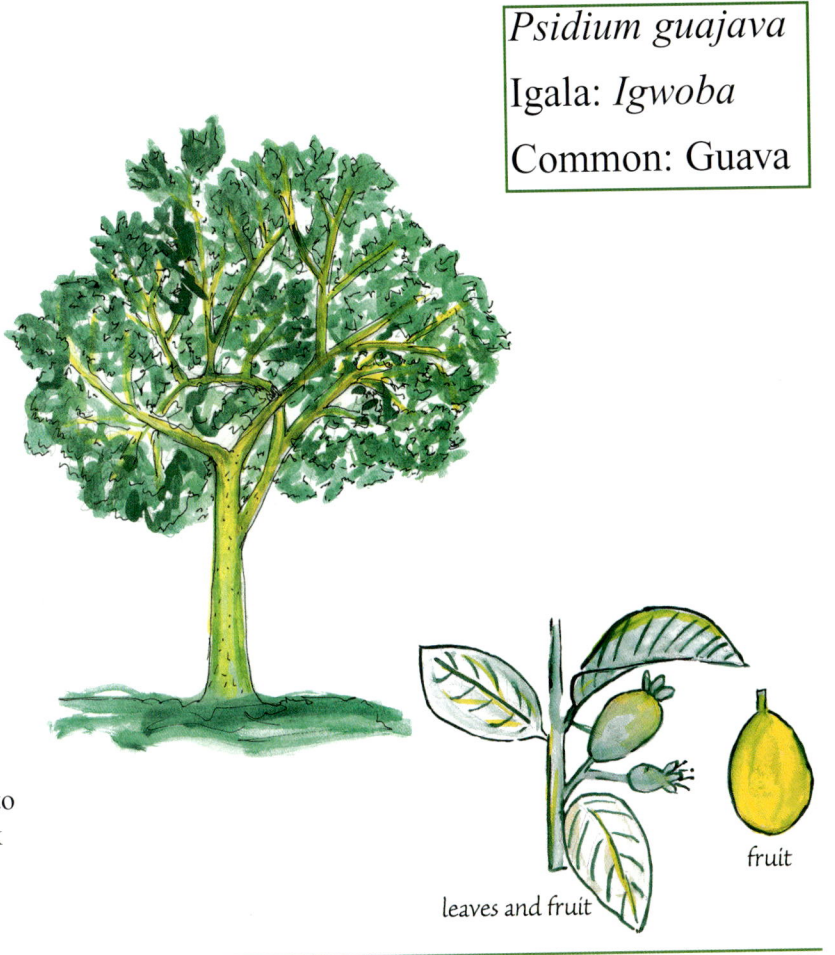

leaves and fruit

fruit

•Food

The ripe fruit serves as a food supplement for morning and afternoon meals.

•Cultural

Has no cultural value.

•Medicinal

The leaves are efficient in the treatment of health disorders especially dysentery in adults when boiled with mango leaves together with the leaves and bark of rose wood. The drink is taken while still warm. Dosage for adults: 1 glass 3 times daily for 7 days.

To cure dysentery in a baby 6 months and over, guava and *ijili* leaves are boiled and added to a porridge to be eaten by the child when hungry.

To cure typhoid, guava leaves are boiled with those of mango, paw paw, acacia, and almond tree. Dosage: 1 glass three times daily for 7 days.

•Other uses

Women use it as fuelwood when trees are old and no longer bearing fruit. Young trees are not cut because of the high value of their fruit and their wood for tools.

Due to the difficulty in obtaining a large straight trunk, the wood is unsuitable for making furniture.

Some guava trees produce forked sticks and are therefore important for building local houses, such as *atakpas*, kitchens, *achakwu* (tombs), along with frames for local mud houses, hoes, cutlasses and axe handles.

Its produces lots of biomass which decomposes easily.

Because of its good shade, women process farm produce beneath its shadow. Men and children play local games there at the end of the day's work.

Its fruits, tools and seedlings have a high market value. The fruits are perishable which limits their economic value. Birds, especially weaverbirds, like the fruits and this makes them more perishable. However, the birds also help propagate this tree, which is an advantage.

Leaves and bark are eaten by goats, but the tree suffers as a consequence.

Pterocarpus erinaceus

Igala: *Ache*

Common: Barwood, Kino

flower

seed

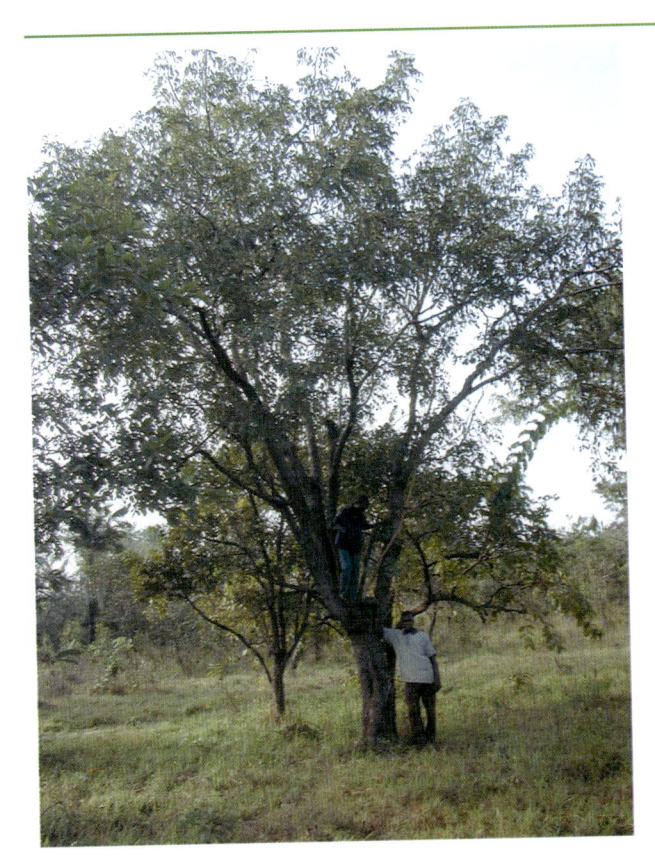

leaves

Family: *Papilionaceae*
A tree that grows up to 40 to 50 ft high. Often covered with golden-yellow flowers when leafless.

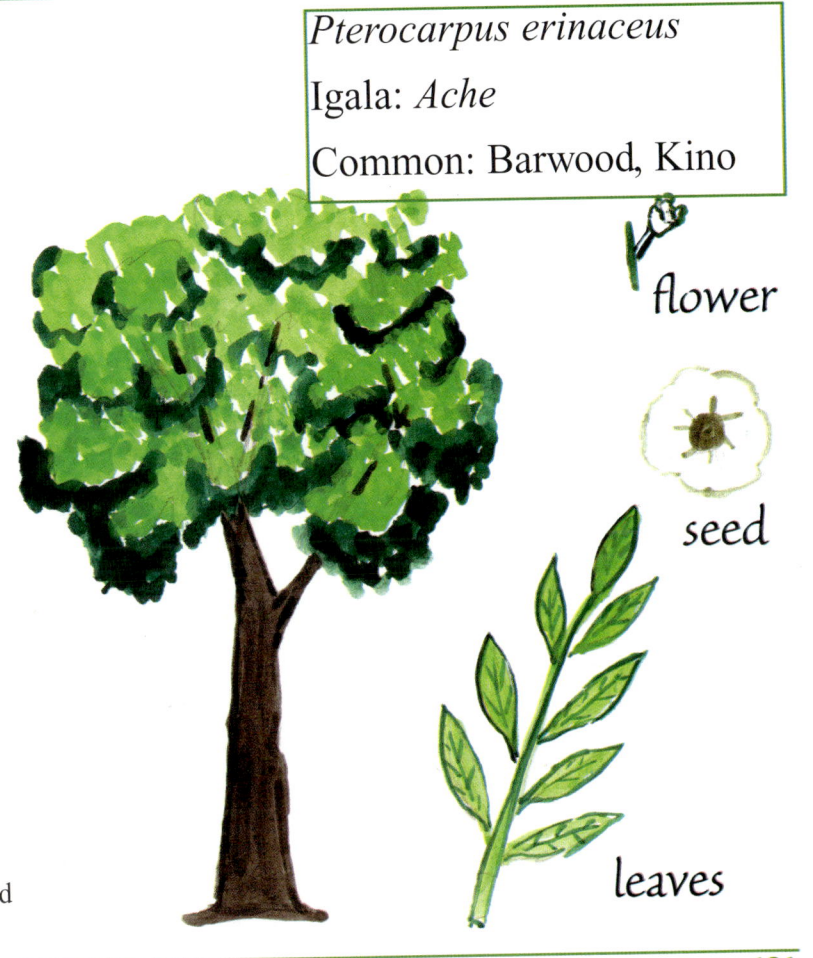

•Food

Not used for food.

•Medicinal

Its leaves when boiled are used for the treatment of toothache and stomach pain. Cooking the leaves and bathing infants in the water while still warm cures oedema.

To cure painful or black menstruation, grind *ache* bark to a paste and add water. Dosage: 1 glass 3 times daily for 7 days.

•Cultural

Artists craft images for idol worshippers from this wood.

A blacksmith constructing farm tools using *Ache* wood for handles.

•Other uses

This tree is on the endangered list and therefore expensive, but when available has many uses.

Renowned as an excellent firewood it is now rarely used for this purpose.

As a hard wood it is used for making paddles, pestles and mortars, seats, local houses, including granaries and *atakpas*, as well as handles for cutlasses, hoes and axes. Tools from this wood are sought-after and fetch a good price. Branches are mostly used as a staking sticks on yam fields.

Only on farms is it used as shade. The trunk and leaves are beautiful and it has many branches. Its leaves rot easily and are a good provider of biomass.

Cattle consume its leaves.

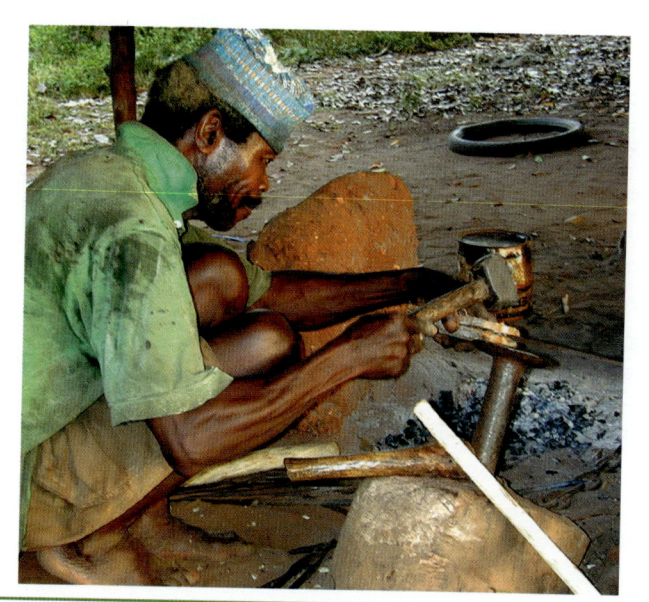

Pterocarpus santalinoides

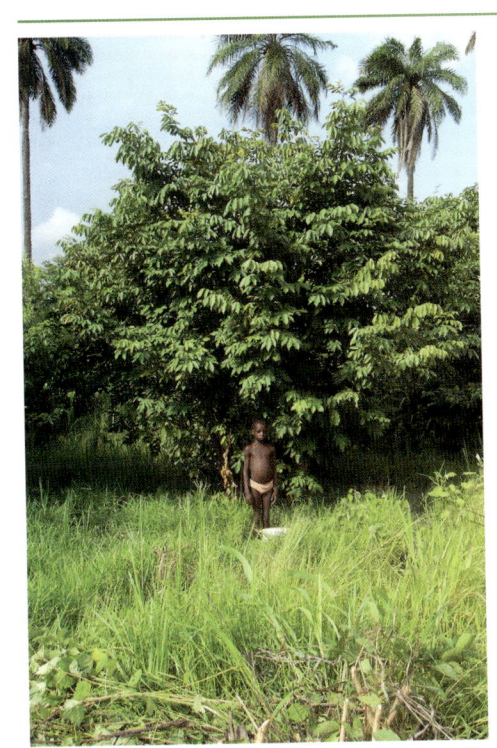

Igala: *Igbẹgbẹ*

Common: Rosewood

leaves

Family: *Papilionaceae*

A tree growing up to 30 to 40 ft tall, but often with a short or divided trunk. Flowers are brilliant yellow. Usually evergreen but can be deciduous. Often found on river banks.

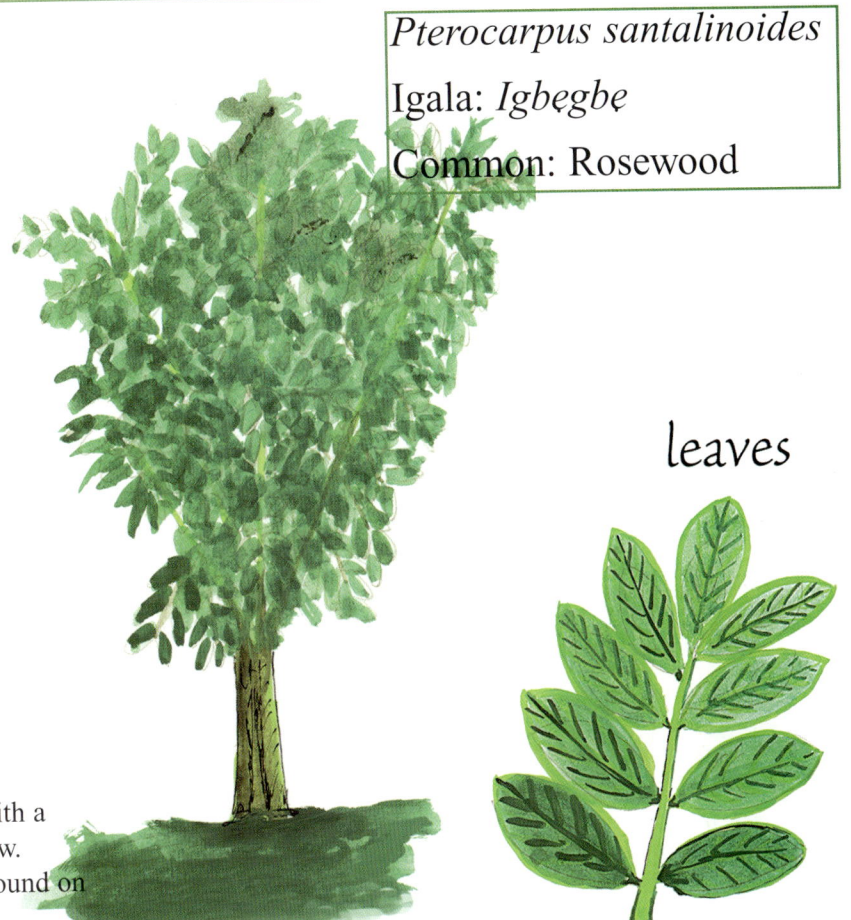

• Food

The fruit and leaves are edible, their popularity confined to the riverine areas.

• Medicinal

It is used mainly for the treatment of dysentery in adults and children.

The bark is boiled with the bark of Ọtọchị (*Mitragyna inermis*) and the root of *obanagbo*. A glass of this medicine is taken 3 times daily for adults, half a glass daily for children.

• Cultural

Artists use it for carving.

• Other uses

Excellent firewood and, though endangered in the plateau areas of the region, it is still enjoyed as firewood in the riverine areas.

Its wood is widely used for small canoes and paddles by local fishermen, despite a short life span of 5 years.

Fishermen use it to support raphia palm leaves for fencing rivers, and also for making handles of spears and fishing-hooks. The paddles, canoes, leaves, bark and seedlings are sources of income.

Its forked sticks are used for building local houses, granaries and *atakpas*. The wood is also used for making handles for farm implements (hoes, cutlasses and axes).

Excellent for soil fertility, and control of some weeds.

Its shade lasts all year, while its yellow flowers and pretty leaves add beauty wherever it grows.

Cattle like to eat its leaves. They also enjoy the bark, which, when over-chewed, results in death for the tree.

Raphia sp.

Igala: *Ẹkpẹ-Ugala, Ẹkpẹ-Ofolo*

Common: Raphia palm

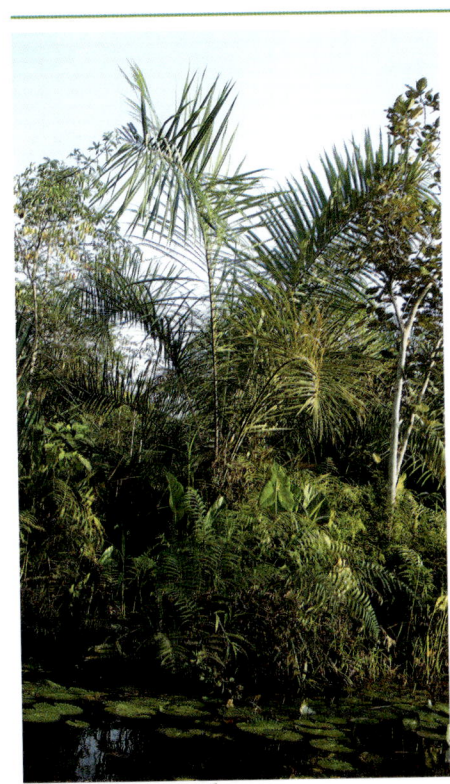

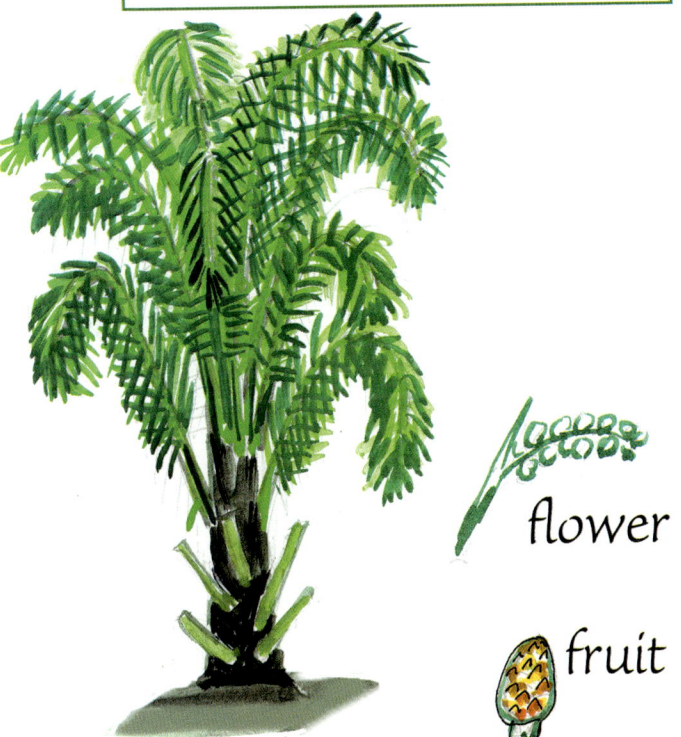

leaf-frond

flower

fruit

Family: *Palmae*

Raphia sp. is a term which covers a number of different species but all are palms of watery places. They grow to a moderate height (25 to 30 ft) and are used for a variety of purposes.

135

•Food

Nothing is edible, but raphia palm is used to produce beverages.

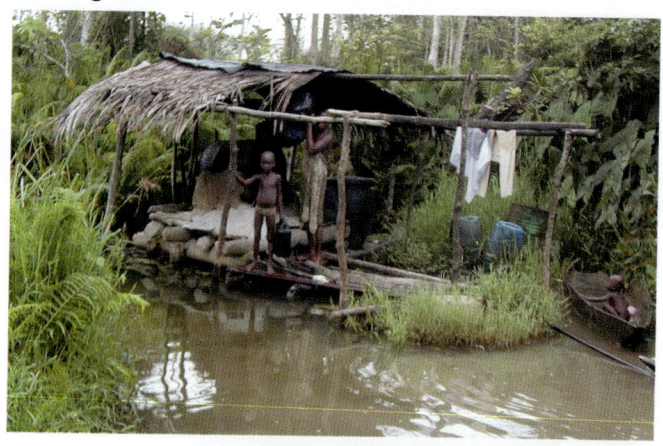

Distilling the wine into *ogogoro* takes place in the swamp where raphia grows.

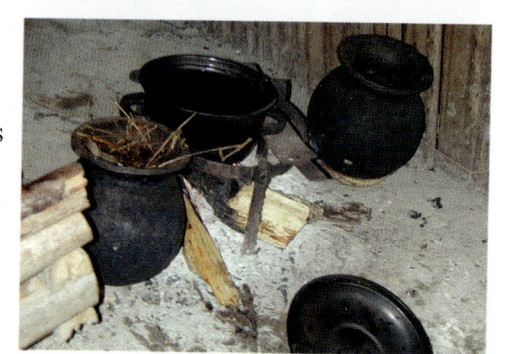

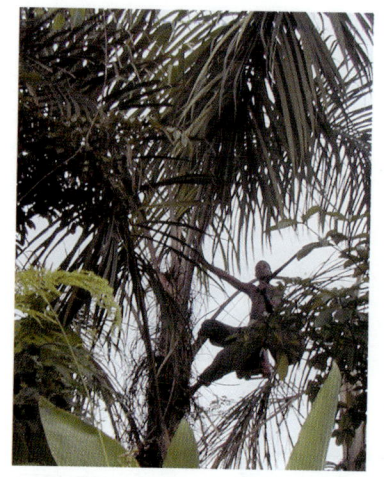

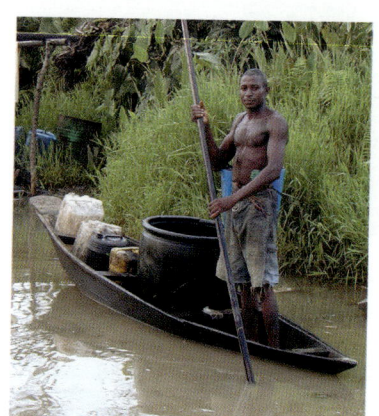

Hard work in difficult conditions

Climbing the raphia tree to tap the 'wine' (sap). A dangerous activity and one only for the skilled.

Delivery of the final product to customers – first by boat, then by bike.

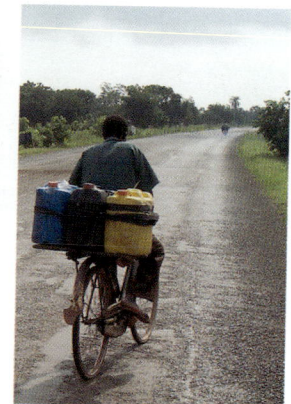

•Medicinal

Raphia wine is the basic ingredient in all medicines for the treatment of poison.

Because its yeast content, it is considered best for eye problems and especially conjunctivitis (locally referred to as Apollo Eye as there was something of a mini-epidemic during the Apollo space missions of the 1960s and early 1970s).

Rubbed onto the skin it helps a measles rash to emerge more quickly, thereby bringing relief to the child.

The local gin (*ogogoro*) is suitable as a disinfectant in laboratories, hospitals and local bathrooms.

It cures backache when added to *inale* root and applied externally.

For the treatment of stomach ache and all fevers *ogogoro* is added to *Ogẹlẹ* stem (neem), which is broken into small pieces and placed in a bottle with the gin.

Dosage: 1 small glass 3 times daily for 7 days.

The *ogogoro*, if added to *ota* root, helps men with ejaculation problems if taken at bedtime.

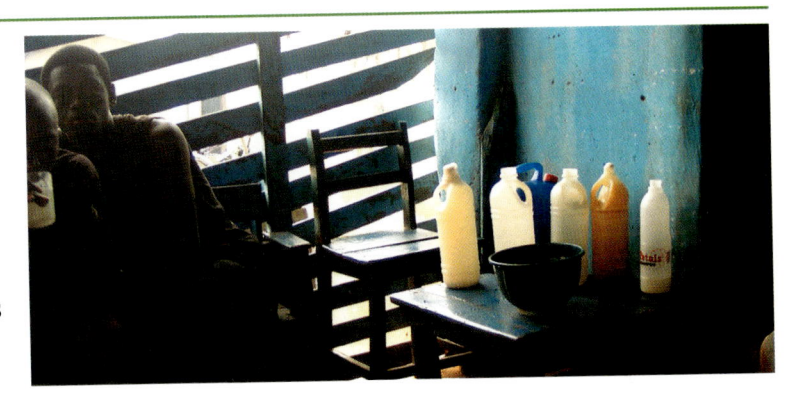

It is believed that people are not vulnerable to cutlass attacks or wounds from similar implements if they drink a mixture of *ogogoro* and a combination of many other roots. However, details of the mixtures are closely guarded secrets.

Mix *ogogoro* with corn porridge and lemon to treat diarrhoea. All ingredients are mixed and 1 spoonful taken 3 times daily for 7 days. In cases of severe problems, the mixture can be used with 2 capsules of tetracycline (an antibiotic). This gives immediate relief, but the treatment has to be monitored carefully.

•Cultural

Wedding ceremonies or significant feasts are not complete without raphia wine. Tradition holds it is the only one acceptable to the ancestors and therefore used in worshipping idols.

For the settlement of community or clan disputes, raphia wine is always recommended as entertainment for the adjudicators. Cola is first brought with the wine and offered to the god of the land before and after a settlement. Raphia wine then serves as the restitution by the offender for his/her crime against the community – for example, someone found stealing or a woman caught in adultery.

The age grade and youth meetings use it for their entertainment, and traditional work groups share it among group members along with *ogogoro* as an appreciation of cooperation. It also helps them to work well and finally relax when tasks are completed.

Igala society is highly organized in terms of allocating tasks relating to the wellbeing of the community, and set aside special days for such negotiations. Raphia wine is central to these occasions and less expensive than palm wine as it yields greater quantities of wine than oil palm.

At the beginning of the fishing season fishermen offer it as sacrifice to the water gods to invoke their blessing for an abundant fish harvest.

A prospective house builder in need of a plot on which to build his house first approaches the chief by offering him raphia palm wine. Negotiations are impossible without this gesture.

Worship sites are normally fenced with raphia.

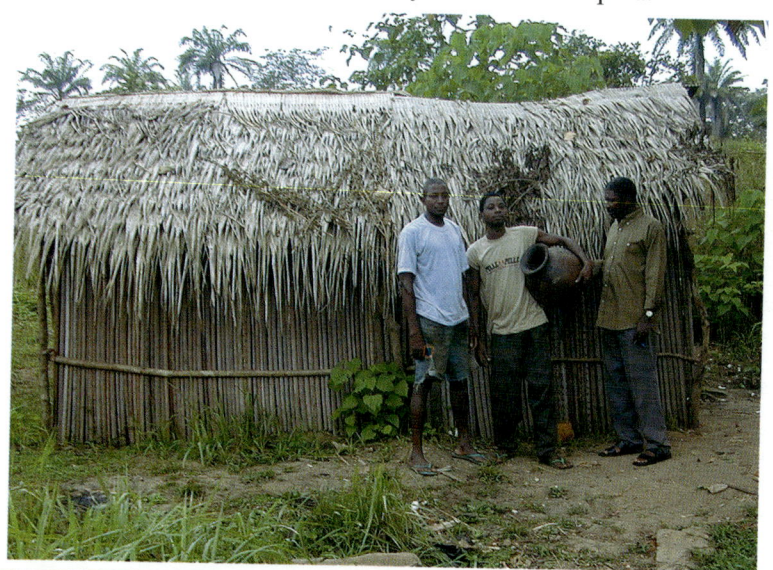

•Other uses

Not many trees can compete with raphia or oil palm in terms of the number of direct products and by-products made from it. The raphia palm is as versatile as the oil palm for the nutrients it supplies to the soil, regardless of whether it is dead or alive.

Every part of the dead tree is used for firewood. It lights quickly and generates a good flame.

Its fibrous stem is used to make local beds, seats, chairs and tables, fans and *atakpas*. Even the reception desks in local hotels are made from it.

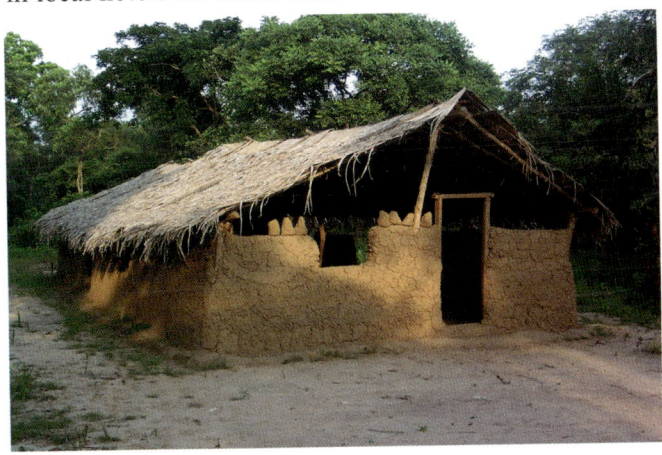

School with a raphia roof

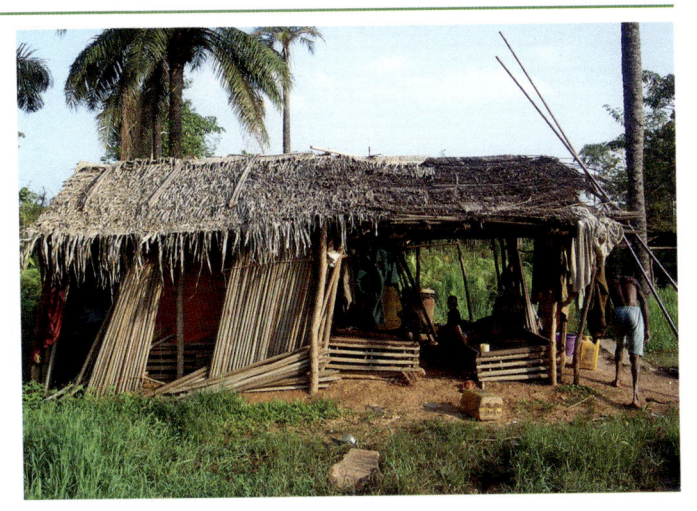

The list is not yet complete. Add grain and yam granaries, stalls for domestic animals and poultry, paddles, fishing materials, bird cages, and guards placed around newly planted seedlings, such as oil palms and oranges, to protect them from cattle.

Every part of this tree has a function in local construction business. Its leaves are used for roofing, and form part of the framework before plastering. Everything in the house, with the exception of the clay, is made from raphia, including doors and windows.

Raphia leaves are also of great importance in marking the boundaries of fishing territories. Each clan has its own site within the river, and raphia leaves control the movement of fish between these sites.

During the floods the various ponds within the Niger river are stocked with fish. When the floods subside, fishermen prevent the fish from moving from these ponds back into the river by using raphia leaves.

These are so skillfully woven that they allow only the water to flow through, but not the fish.

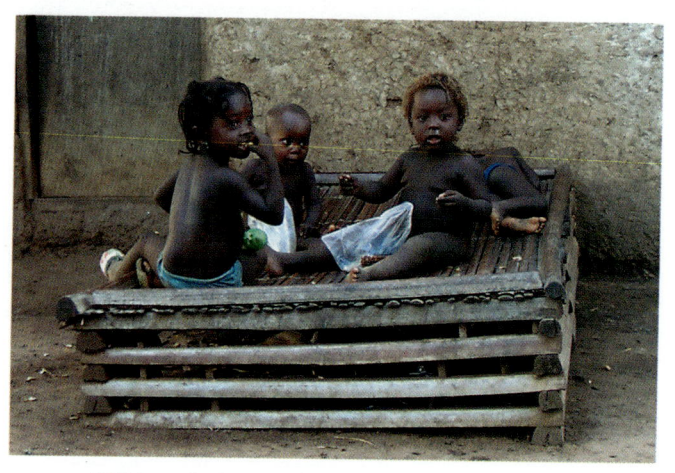

Children playing on a bed made from raphia fronds.

Raphia leaves used in drying fish ensure easier and more thorough curing. Even the flat baskets where fish are displayed in the market are made from raphia leaves. They are also used for staking yams.

Fans and brooms made from raphia are durable and therefore popular with housewives particularly during the hot season and *harmattan* (dry desert winds). Traditional dancers use them to adorn their bodies during festivals.

Every part of this tree sells well in the market. The wine is transported to the market by the men and sold wholesale to women. The women then retail it to consumers.

Local entrepreneurs producing fans, beds, brooms, paddles and thatching services use raphia palm as their raw material. The hot drink (*ogogoro*), which is one of its main by-products, provides a source of income for many women who engage in this industry. Wives of tappers also usually benefit from their husband's work.

Indirectly it also increases sales of plastic containers for those who earn a living in this way.

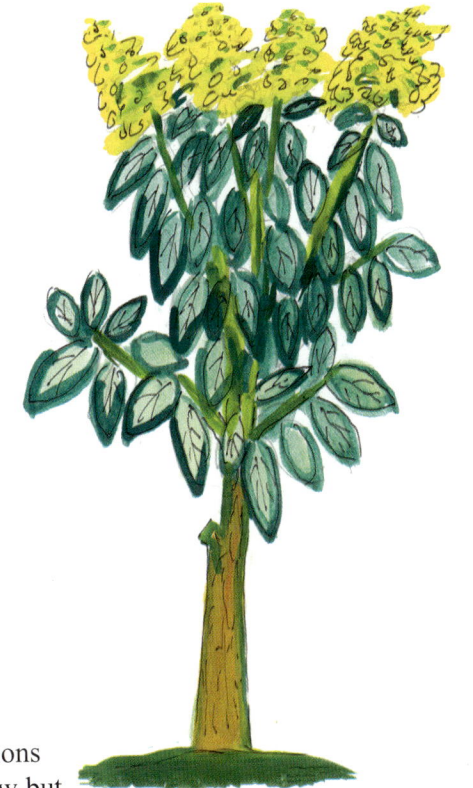

Tectona grandis

Igala: *Oli-are*

Common: Teak

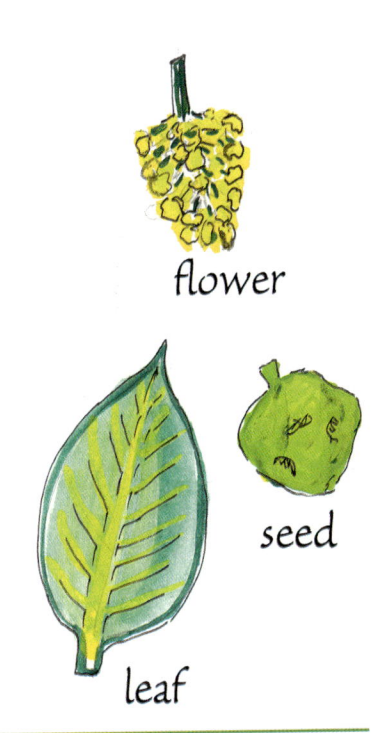

flower

seed

leaf

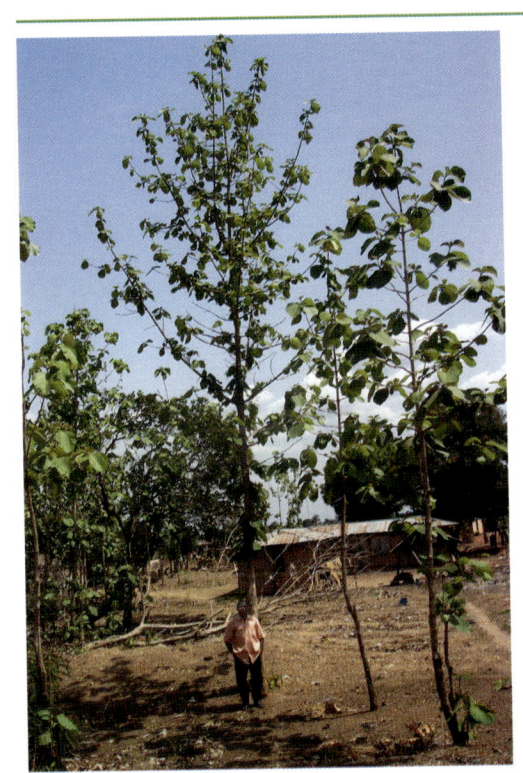

Family: *Verbenaceae*

Native to Asia but now widely grown in plantations across the tropics. Heartwood dark golden yellow but turns a dark brown following exposure to air. Widely used for construction.

141

- **Food**

No value as food.

- **Medicinal**

For medicinal purposes its tender reddish leaf is prepared to treat anaemia and typhoid fever.

- **Cultural**

No cultural value.

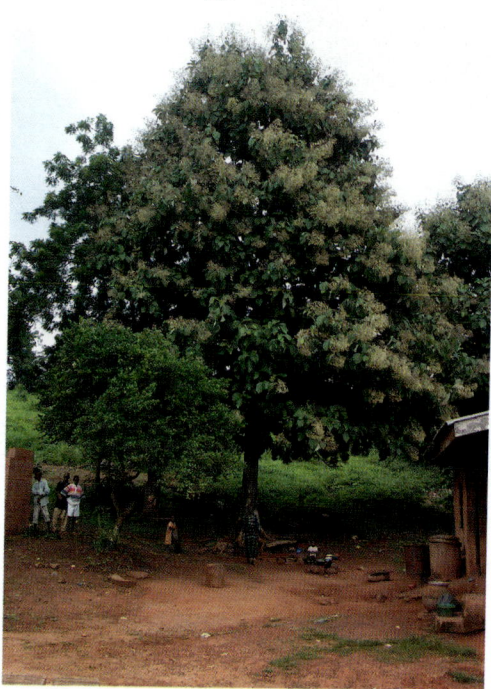

- **Other uses**

Farmer-friendly in every way, teak is fast growing and will re-grow up to 10 times after cutting, involving little labour. Housewives collect parts of the tree left over after sawing as it lasts long in the fire.

Now popular for furniture of all kinds, it is said to 'have a good face', responding well to a coat of varnish; if sandpapered, 'designs' (grain) appear.

Though fast growing, it is durable and has resistance to woodworm, its straight trunk making it acceptable to carpenters. A good source of income, it has gained a place in the export market.

Locally, teak is used for lorry backs and floors, roofing, electric poles, granaries, pillars and frames for local houses, axe and cutlass handles. Hoe handles are rarely made out of it as it does not produce a forked stick.

Teak is famous for its biomass even if its leaves are slow to decompose. Because they are extra large they are useful for controlling weeds and last long as mulch. Because of their large size they can be sold in the market to those preserving cola nuts.

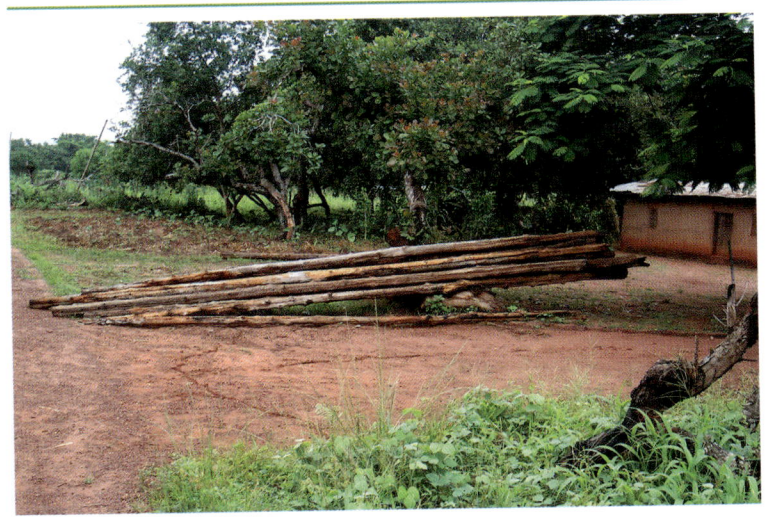

Teak poles to be used for a rural electrification project. These are normally treated to protect them against termite attack.

Wooden poles are being replaced with more expensive concrete structures for such projects.

A forest or plantation of teak has a cooling effect on the atmosphere.

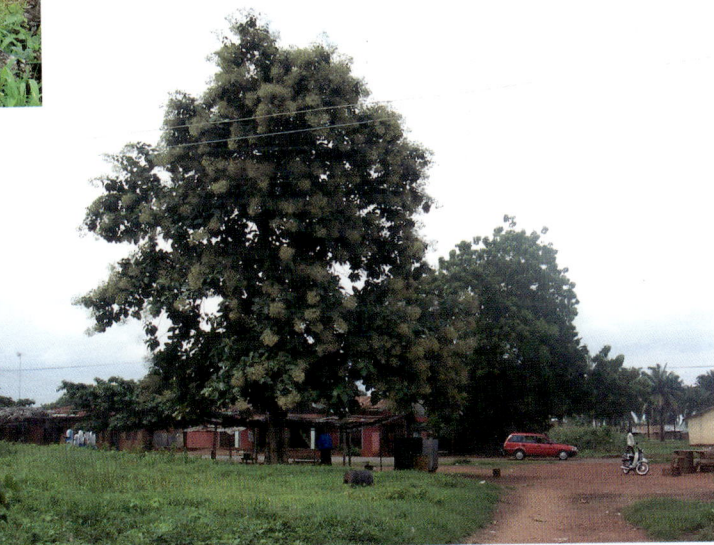

143

Treculia Africana

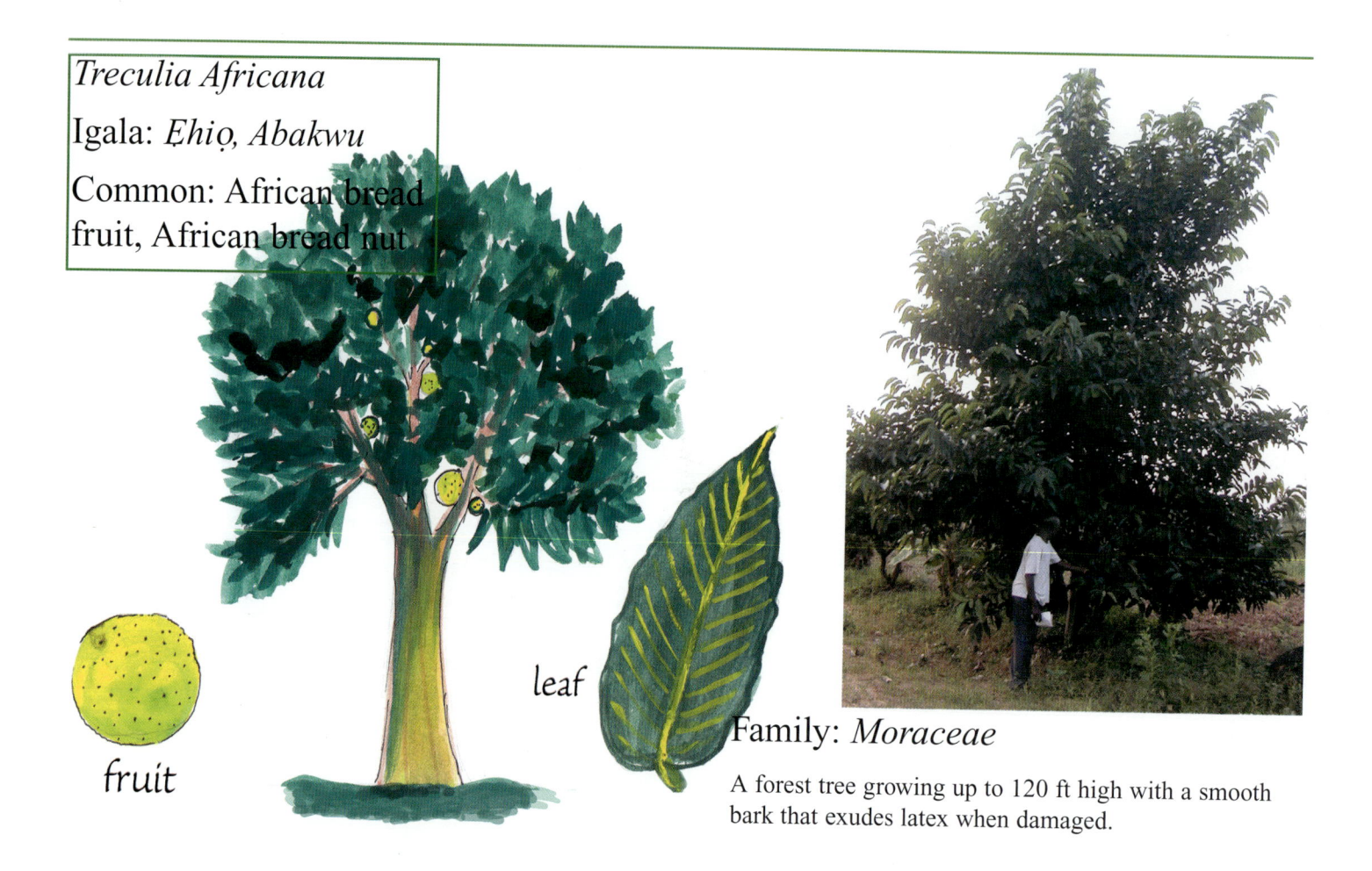

Igala: *Ehio, Abakwu*

Common: African bread fruit, African bread nut

fruit

leaf

Family: *Moraceae*

A forest tree growing up to 120 ft high with a smooth bark that exudes latex when damaged.

•Food

Rich in protein, it can be cooked in many ways. The preparation of seeds is however lengthy and similar to that of other local beans which are dried and preserved. Seeds sell well as a cash crop.

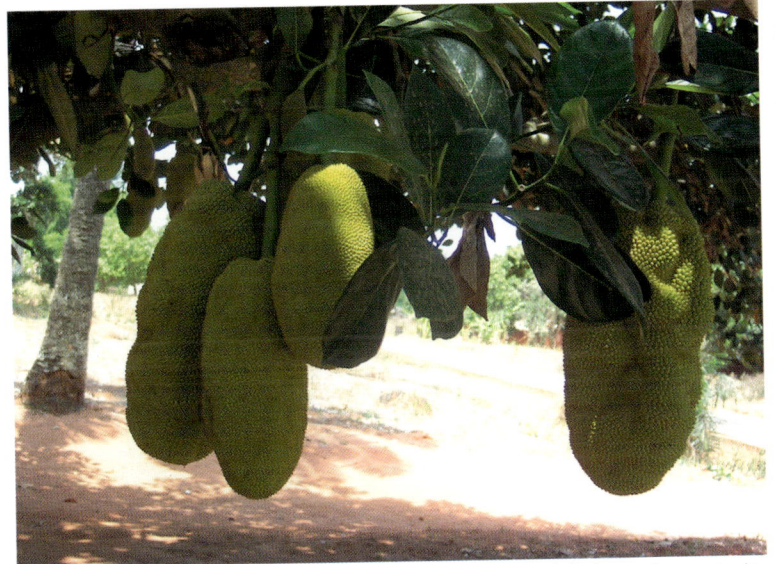

Bread fruit nearing maturity

•Medicinal

The bark when boiled is used for diabetics. One glass is taken daily for as long as necessary.

•Cultural

Although grown in this region for many years, it is only recently its uses are becoming better known. This is thanks to nutrition clinics, women's programmes and interchange between ethnic groups who have relied on it as a staple for many years. Yet another example of cultural exchange.

•Other uses

Though not generally used for firewood, if available people are happy to use it.

Breadfruit wood is used mainly for granaries, handles for cutlasses, hoes and axes.

Even if its leaves do not compose easily, they eventually produce good biomass.

Despite growing on the lower branches, the fruit is so heavy it can kill or injure a person upon falling. The tree is therefore not suitable for shade, and to avoid casualties is not grown near compounds.

The tree itself looks elegant.

Animals like to eat its fruit and leaves.

Vitex doniana

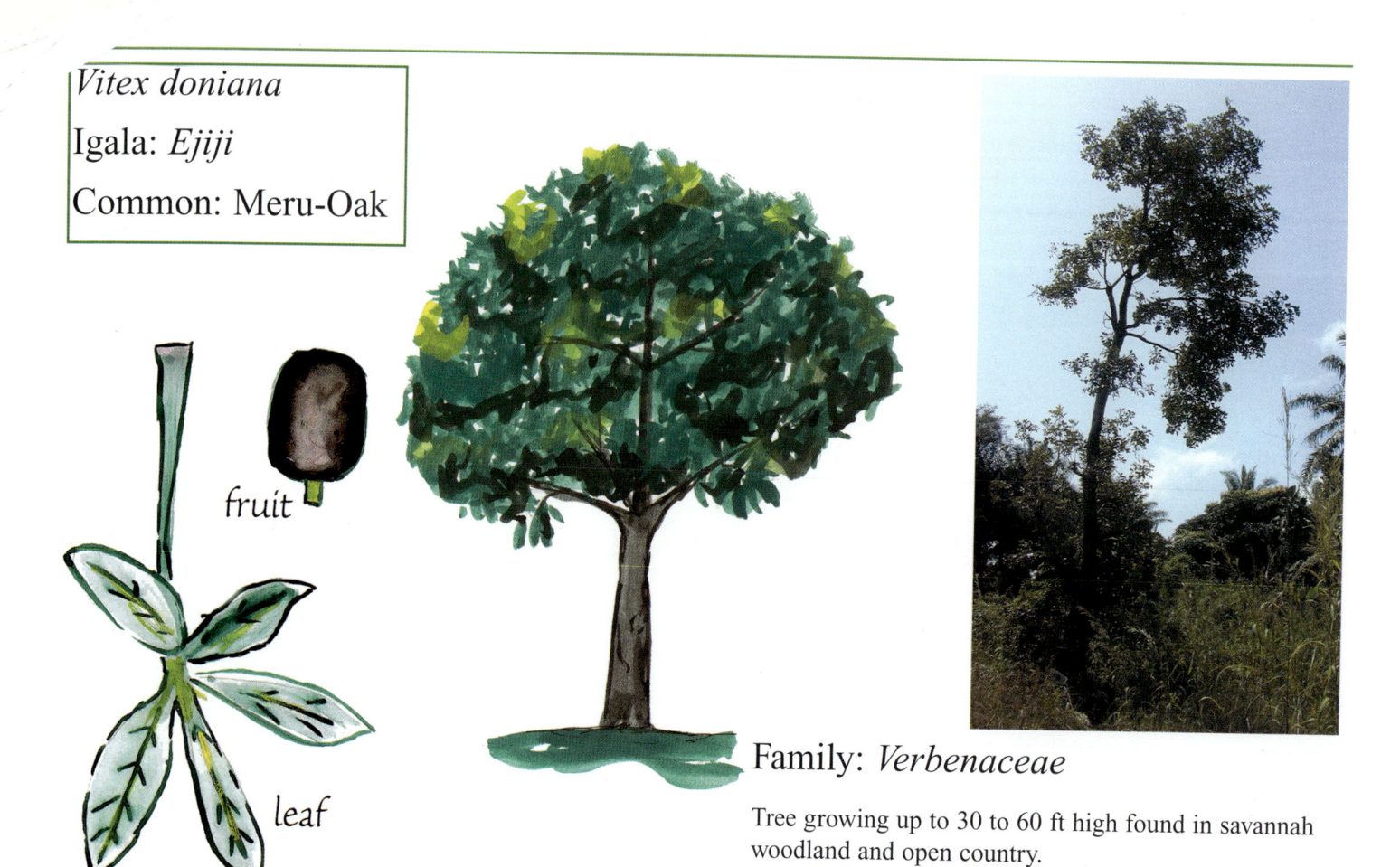

Igala: *Ejiji*

Common: Meru-Oak

fruit

leaf

Family: *Verbenaceae*

Tree growing up to 30 to 60 ft high found in savannah woodland and open country.

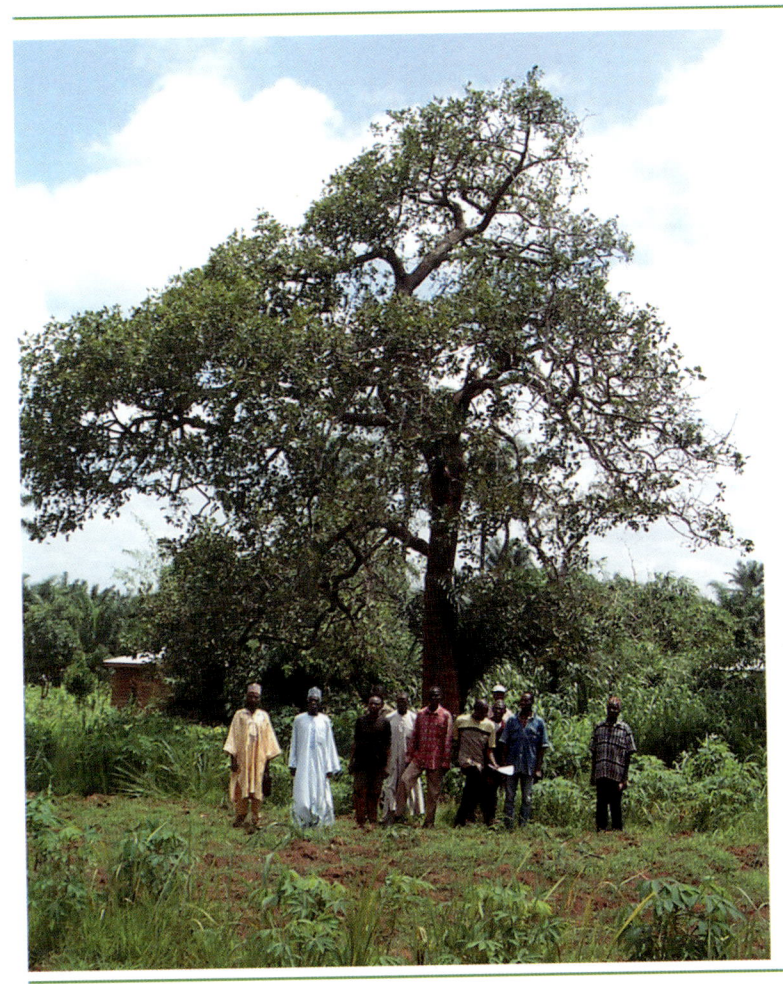

•Food

The leaves, fruit and liquid from the fruit are highly valued in the diet. Fruits are eaten raw and can be processed to oil which tastes like honey.

•Cultural

Artists like the pliable soft wood for carving. Even if it stays for years in the sun the wood does not crack.

Moslems use it as ink when writing their *rubutu* on slates.

•Medicinal

The tree is very friendly to young mothers: its leaves and skin are boiled, and the warmed liquid used for bathing premature babies. A tiny drop can be given to the baby on a spoon 3 times daily.

Fever and anaemia can be treated with the same formulation, the liquid taken 3 times daily. The leaves are used to cure anaemia and prepared in the form of vegetable soup.

To cure stomach ache for a mother who has newly delivered, boil the bark of *ejiji* and drink the extract. Dosage: 1 glass 3 times a day for 7 days.

•Other uses

Besides producing excellent firewood that lasts for days, until the dry wood completely disappears, it also has many uses including the manufacture of domestic and office furniture, canoes, paddles, local seats, pestles, farm tool handles, frame work for *atakpas*, granaries, dwelling houses and stalls for cattle, as well as a traditional game (known as *ichę*).

Its ash is used for plastering local houses and in local soap production. The Hausa bow is also constructed from it.

The liquid processed from its fruits looks like honey and used to supplement local dishes such as porridge and other corn dishes. This liquid is now very valuable in local markets and known as *ejiji*. A pint bottle costs about 2 dollars which is considered very expensive.

The leaves are sold for vegetable soup. They also decompose easily and under every tree is found *awolowo* grass (*Eupatorium odoratum*), a sure indicator of both good soil and moisture content.

Leaves have a special brown hue, which make it distinctive from the other trees especially at the commencement of the rainy season. Animals and fowl eat the leaves when young.

Every household aims at having this tree as it gives shade and food all year round, and the housewife does not have to travel for her family's favourite ingredients.

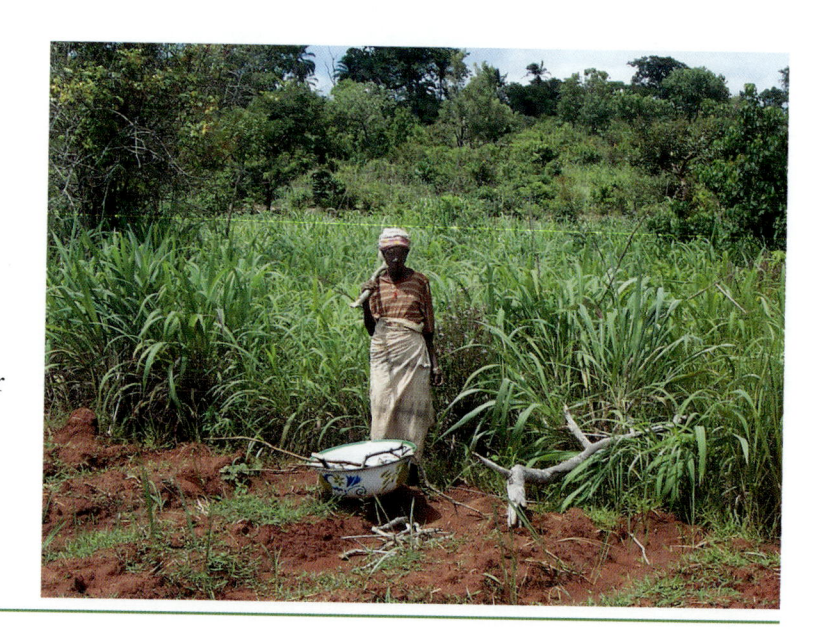

Index

Abakwu	144
Abo	92
Ache	131
Achęchę	66
Adansonia digitata	1
African Border Tree	113
African bread fruit	144
African bread nut	144
African cherry	29
African Copaiba	50
African locust bean	116
Afzelia africana	5
Agba	50
Agirigele	52
Ago	85
Agwu	23
Agwugwu	23
Akpachi	50
Alemu	32
Alemu-Hajalini	35
Anacardiaceae	10, 95, 101
Annacardium occidentale	10
Anthocleista nobilis	13
Anwa	5
Apocynaceae	92
Atala	46
Aubrevillea kerstingii	16
Avocado	119
Ayigęlę	52
Azadiracta indica	19
Balsam Tree	50
Baobab	1
Barwood	131
Bignoniaceae	89, 113
Bombacaceae	1, 23
Bombax costatum	23
Bonko fruit	110
Bush mango	80
Cabbage Tree	13
Caesalpiniaceae	5, 48, 50, 52
Cam wood	5
Carica papaya	26
Caricaceae	26
Cashew	10
Chinese banyan	70
Chrysophyllum albidum	29
Citrus aurantium	32
Citrus x tangelo	35
Coconut	37
Cocus Nucifera	37
Cola	40, 43, 46
Cola acuminata	40

Cola gigantea	43
Cola nitida	46
Coral Flower	46
Cynometra vogelii	48
Daniellia oliveri	50
Dialium guineense	52
Ebenebe	43
Ẹbiẹ	89
Echibakpa	26
Echikala	95
Ẹhia	29
Ẹhiọ	144
Ejiji	146
Ekebergia senegalensis	54
Ẹkpẹ	57
Ẹkpẹ-ofolo	135
Ẹkpe-ugala	135
Elaeis Guineensis	57
Ẹnache	77
Erythrina senegalensis	66
Euphorbiaceae	77, 121
Fan palm	123
Ficus capensis	68
Ficus thonningii	70
Fig tree	68
Gmelina	72
Gmelina arborea	72
Guava	129
Hannoa undulata	75
Hog plum	95
Hymenocardia acida	77
Igbẹgbẹ	133
Igogo	95
Igwoba	129
Ikachu	10
Indian laurel	70
Indigo	48
Invingia gabonensis	80
Iroko	104, 108
Iron tree	98
Irvingia wombulu	83
Irvingia Gabonensis	80
Irvingiaceae	80, 83
Kapok tree	23
Khaya senegalensis	85
Kigelia africana	89
Kino	131
Landolphia amoena	92
Lannea nigritana	95
Lauraceae	119
Locust bean	127
Loganiaceae	13
Lophira lanceolata	98
Mahogany	85

Makarara	121	Ogbu	70
Malayan banyan	70	Ọgẹlẹ	110
Mangifera indica	101	Ogichi	113
Mango	101	Ogirichi	113
Meliaceae	19, 54, 85	Oil palm	57
Meru-Oak	146	Okopi	98
Millicia excelsa	104	Okpehie	126
Mimosaceae	16, 116, 126	Okpuye	126
Miombo Red-Heart	77	Okra tree	83
Mitragyna inermis	108	Oli-are	141
Moraceae	68, 70, 144	Oli-Ọda	19
Morinda lucida	110	Orachi	54
Myrtaceae	129	Orange	32
Neem	19	Ọro-Ayikpẹlẹ	83
Newbouldia laevis	113	Ọro-Egili	80
Obi-Akechi	46	Ọtọchi	108
Obi-Igala	40	Palmae	38, 57, 123, 135
Obobo	1	Papilionaceae	66, 104, 131, 133
Ochnaceae	98	Parkia biglobosa	116
Ọda	70	Pawpaw	26
Ọda/Ogbu	70	Persea americana	119
Ode	121	Phyllanthus discoides	121
Odo	123	Podococcus barteri	123
Odobala	75	Prosopsis africana	126
Odogwu	13	Psidium guajava	129
Odologwu	13	Pterocarpus erinaceus	131
Ọgbaikolo	68	Pterocarpus santalinoides	133

151

Raphia palm	135
Raphia sp.	135
Rosewood	133
Rubiaceae	110
Rutaceae	32, 35
Sapotaceae	29
Sausage tree	89
Simaroubaceae	75
Sterculiaceae	40, 43, 46
Tangerine	35
Teak	141
Tectona grandis	141
Treculia africana	144
Ube Agiliki	119
Udu	16
Ugba	116
Ugbakolo	68
Ugo	43
Uli	48
Uloko	104
Ulomu	32
Umagolo	101
Umopula	75
Unọba	37
Unya	89
Uri	48
Uroko	104
Utẹ	29
Utiẹ	29
Velvet Tamarind	52
Verbenaceae	72, 141, 146
Vitex doniana	146
West African Gum Copal	50